Clinical Data Quality Checks for CDISC Compliance Using SAS

Clinical Data Quality Checks for CDISC Compliance Using SAS

Sunil Gupta

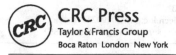

CRC Press
Taylor & Francis Group
Boca Raton London New York

CRC Press is an imprint of the
Taylor & Francis Group, an **informa** business
A CHAPMAN & HALL BOOK

CRC Press
Taylor & Francis Group
6000 Broken Sound Parkway NW, Suite 300
Boca Raton, FL 33487-2742

© 2020 by Taylor & Francis Group, LLC
CRC Press is an imprint of Taylor & Francis Group, an Informa business

No claim to original U.S. Government works

Printed on acid-free paper

International Standard Book Number-13: 978-0-367-36278-2 (Hardback)
978-0-367-36277-5 (Paperback)

Library of Congress Cataloging-in-Publication Data

Names: Gupta, Sunil, 1963- author.
Title: Clinical data quality checks for CDISC compliance using SAS / by
    Sunil Gupta.
Description: Boca Raton, FL : Taylor & Francis, [2020] | Includes bibliographical references and
    index. | Summary: "This book helps you create a system of SDTM and ADaM checks that can
    be tracked for continuous improvement. How often have you encountered issues such as
    missing required variables, duplicate records, invalid derived variables and invalid sequence
    of two dates? With the SAS programming techniques introduced in this book, you can start to
    monitor these and more complex data and CDISC compliance issues. With increased
    standardization in SDTM and ADaM specifications and data values, codelist dictionaries can
    be created for better organization, planning and maintenance. This book includes a SAS
    program to create excel files containing unique values from all SDTM and ADaM variables as
    columns. In addition, another SAS program compares SDTM and ADaM codelist dictionaries
    with codelists from define.xml specifications. Having tools to automate this process greatly
    saves time from doing it manually"-- Provided by publisher.
Identifiers: LCCN 2019023651 (print) | LCCN 2019023652 (ebook) | ISBN 9780367362775
    (paperback) | ISBN 9780367362782 (hardback) | ISBN 9780429345043 (ebook)
Subjects: LCSH: SAS (Computer file) | Medical care--Standards--United
    States. | Medical care--United States--Quality control.
Classification: LCC QA276.45.S27 G87 2020 (print) | LCC QA276.45.S27
    (ebook) | DDC 005.5/5--dc23
LC record available at https://lccn.loc.gov/2019023651
LC ebook record available at https://lccn.loc.gov/2019023652

Visit the Taylor & Francis Web site at
http://www.taylorandfrancis.com

and the CRC Press Web site at
http://www.crcpress.com

Contents

Preface

Clinical Data Quality Checks for CDISC Compliance Using SAS is a concise guide to help you apply innovative SAS programming techniques for improving data quality and CDISC compliance. The book capitalizes on these topics for more effective management.

- Manage controlled terminology dictionaries

- Monitor and better understand Pinnacle 21 issues

- Control and customize CDISC compliance checks

- Leverage metadata for automation

- QA checklists for better FDA submissions

Managing controlled terminology dictionaries involves automatically creating SDTM and ADaM codelist dictionaries without manually running Proc FREQ on each SDTM and ADaM variable. In addition, tools to automatically compare SDTM and ADaM codelist dictionaries with define.xml specification codelists help to quickly identify differences in codelists so that define.xml files are correctly represented.

Monitoring and understanding Pinnacle 21 issues are essential for SAS programmers in the pharmaceutical industry. Most SAS programmers use Pinnacle 21 Community or Enterprise versions to check for CDISC compliance. This book reviews the main components of the Pinnacle 21 Enterprise version – SDTM/ADaM compliance, SDTM/ADaM repository, define.xml and control terms and value-level metadata. This book also shows examples of the five channels of CDISC compliance issues – unit level, multiple variables and datasets, new variables, protocol compliance and metadata and data transfer metrics.

This book has tools to jumpstart controlling and customizing CDISC compliance checks. Below are key features:

- Level of checks to apply
  - SDTMs and ADaMs vitals
  - SDTMs and ADaMs data
  - CDISC specifications compliance
  - CDISC data compliance
  - Protocol compliance
  - Codelist dictionary compliance
- When to apply checks
  - Database acceptance lock
  - SDTMs and ADaMs refresh
  - Snapshot analysis
- Different checks for different customers
  - Site management
  - Data management
  - SAS programmers
  - Statisticians

Leveraging metadata for automation requires advanced SAS programming skills to dynamically access and process a directory of files, such as SAS datasets or SAS programs, so that no hard coding is required. SAS tools include LIBNAME, DATA step, SAS macro programming, SAS and dataset functions, Proc SQL, Proc COMPARE and Proc MEANS. Many standard and custom metadata such as # and type variables, maximum variable length and descriptive statistics on categorical and continuous variables can be created to manage the quality of data.

With each FDA submission, QA checklists assure all items are completed and validated. The book includes four practical QA checklists for SDTM and ADaM mapping, clinical study milestones, Pinnacle 21 issues and Pinnacle 21 define specifications to define.XML. The SDTM and ADaM mapping checklist includes examples of macros that many organizations have to perform common functions. The clinical study milestones checklist includes items in the database lock process. Both Pinnacle 21 checklists confirm key compliance levels.

Acknowledgments

A s I complete the final review of Clinical Data Quality Checks for CDISC Compliance using the SAS book, I am reminded of fond memories of being in the pharmaceutical and medical device industries for over 25 years and the passion I have had to improve data quality and strive for higher standards. For each project I have supported, data quality checks were just as important as primary and secondary safety and efficacy analysis. This book is a result of all my long hours to push the SAS envelope for more robust and data-driven processes. The unique SAS programming techniques I developed along the way have enabled me to reach my goals as well as enable me to mentor other SAS programmers. In addition, my clients have benefited from the comprehensive checklists I have created to assure all proper steps were followed in FDA submission preparation and execution. I hope you too will find the book and SASSavvy.com invaluable resources. I look forward to hearing your comments about the book.

I would like to thank my wife, Bindiya, and daughters, Aarti and Anupama, for their support, commitment and excitement. I would also like to thank my book reviewers, Linfeng Xu, Paul Gill, Roger DeAngelis and Chris Weiner, for their valuable suggestions to improve the book. Their experience in the industry has helped make the book more practical. This book along with my other four SAS books, *Quick Results with the Output Delivery System*, *Data Management Using the SAS Learning Edition*, *Sharpening Your SAS Skills*, and *Sharpening Your Advanced SAS Skills* has been a dream come true.

Author

Sunil Gupta is an international speaker, bestselling SAS author and a global corporate CDISC trainer. Mr. Gupta is a principal SAS/CDISC consultant and mentor. Most recently, he taught both of his CDISC online classes in conjunction with the University of California at San Diego and SAS® Institute India. New in 2019, he is developing a new class on data science using SAS class. In 2011, he launched his unique SAS resource blog, SASSavvy.com, for smarter SAS searches. Currently, SAS Savvy's membership consists mostly of SAS programmers, university students and pharmaceutical corporate accounts.

In 2018, Mr. Gupta was the Quick Tips section chair at the first PhUSE conference in Raleigh, and in 2016, he was a CDISC oncology ADaM reviewer. In 2013, he was recognized by SAS Institute's Circle of Excellence for 20 years of service. In 2008, he was chosen as one of the '100 Notable People in the Medical Device Industry' for his contributions. Two of his popular pharmaceutical industry leadership articles include 'How Cloud-Based Tools Can Help with FDA Compliance' in the *Life Science Leadership* magazine and 'Standards for Clinical Data Quality and Compliance Checks' in the *Society for Clinical Data Management* and *Pharmaceutical Programming* journals.

Each year, Mr. Gupta has been an invited presenter at many SAS conferences for his 'highly acclaimed' Proc SQL hands-on workshops. In 2018, he was the keynote speaker at the PhUSE SDE International Meeting in Hyderabad, India. He has been using SAS software for over 20 years and is a SAS-based certified professional. He is also the author of *Quick Results with the Output Delivery System, Sharpening Your SAS Skills*, and *Sharpening Your Advanced SAS Skills*.

CHAPTER 1

Overview of Data Quality and Compliance Checks

INTRODUCTION

While the industrywide use of the Pinnacle 21 tool to document CDISC compliance issues is well-known by many pharmaceutical and medical device companies as well as the FDA, successful organizations have gone the extra mile to build in-house compliance checks macros to monitor and manage issue resolutions. The compliance checks in this book serve to complement Pinnacle 21 checks as well as be consistent with them. In addition, this publication has new tools to better manage controlled terminology dictionaries. A key benefit of creating a system of compliance checks in-house is that organizations have more control over of the types and methods to manage data issues. For many organizations, this book fills that void by outlining a roadmap of proven SAS programming and macro techniques. In addition, organizations can customize checks for other purposes, such as database acceptance and locks, confirming unique USUBJIDs, ensuring codelist integrity and creating derived variables. Since metadata is an integral component of the compliance check process, an in-house system assures a higher quality source of data and checks throughout the SDTM and ADaM creation process. Good clinical practices suggest that organizations should leverage metadata for more study-based rules, address common issues and create more data-driven automated processing for quicker response times. With this approach, organizations can scale up to handle more studies with minimal increase in technical staff.

The importance of data quality and compliance checks to the overall integrity and outcome of clinical studies cannot be over emphasized. It is imperative that all organizations supporting the collection, organization and analysis of clinical data apply these checks when first receiving the data. This is required to confirm the actual data received is as expected. Finally, any data transformations must be verified to assure no change in data integrity.

This chapter provides an overview of level of checks for systemic and detail issues. This applies to the whole clinical cycle when first receiving raw data to the final analysis. This will encompass a variety of types of checks for different customers so that the whole team is actively working toward a quality FDA submission. There are four high-level categories of validation checks: metadata-level checks, value-level checks, logical checks and cross-reference checks. Examples include checking for missing values, range checks, protocol violation checks and checks for duplicates.

Chapters 2 through 7 contain examples of each level check. Many of the sample domains used in this book are from define.xml 2.0 release package 20140424, which uses SDTM IG version 3.2. Many of the examples in this book use the same SAS programming structure logic to create a detailed-level data check dataset called DCA and summary-level data check datasets DCB and DC. DCA dataset saves only the check variables and creates and sets the BAD_VALUE variable to 1 for any failed check. The key to this method is to apply the correct condition to define failed records. The DCB dataset uses summary functions on the DCA dataset to count the number of records with BAD_VALUE = 1. The advantage of this approach is to create an alert at the summary level for any compliance issue as well as have the option to drill down to the detail patient, test name and visit date. You can customize DCA datasets to contain relevant variables from SDTMs as well as the variable order. Often, reviewing only relevant variables, instead of all SDTM variables, facilitates understanding the root cause of the issue sooner. DC dataset contains useful dataset vitals. The intermediate DCA, DCB and DC datasets from each check can be renamed and appended to save all checks into one overall summary dataset. The CDISC compliance check datasets in Figure 1.1 show the relationship of the detail and summary datasets.

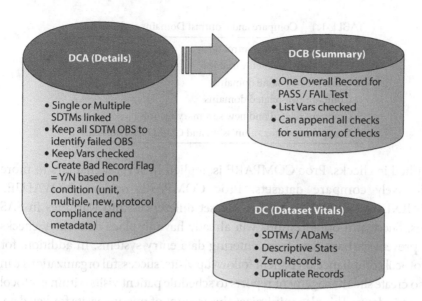

FIGURE 1.1   CDISC compliance check datasets.

See Figure A.1 for general process flow of SAS programs. See Figure A.2 for data model of datasets and key variables. By focusing and being proactive to address potential data and compliance issues, SAS programmers will inherently become expert SAS programmers and more knowledgeable about the eCTD filing process and future industry standards. Join the growing SASSavvy.com community for the latest CDISC and SAS programming tips. Please contact the author at Sunil@SASSavvy.com for a copy of the SAS examples and any SAS programming or CDISC-related questions. All data in this publication is completely fabricated by the author. The output seen in tables and figures is essentially random but tends to be representative of a typical clinical trial. Any resemblance to live data is purely coincidental.

1.1 LEVEL OF CHECKS TO APPLY

By applying checks across all levels in the process to create SDTMs and ADaMs, organizations can better handle the source of data and compliance issues. From systemic issues, which may be corrected with updated SOPs or training, to detail issues from data entry errors, corrective action can be targeted for more immediate impact. Checks can be applied at each level: Dataset, data, protocol compliance, CDISC data compliance and CDISC specifications compliance. The difference between CDISC data and specifications compliance levels are based on data content rules and data structure rules. In Table 1.1, the compare and contrast domains and variables chart shows types of comparisons

TABLE 1.1   Compare and Contrast Domains and Variables

1. Compare data and control terms
2. Compare two related variables
3. Compare two same domains
4. Compare two related domains
5. Compare related and new summary records
6. Compare sponsor submission and CDISC spec domains

applied in checks. Proc COMPARE is applied in several chapters to more effectively compare datasets. Proc COMPARE options, NOVALUES WARNING NOPRINT, convert dataset differences into warnings in SAS logs. Successful organizations will already have in place data entry checks to prevent garbage data from entering data entry systems. In addition, for protocol compliance on patient follow-up visits, successful organizations can also create site management reports to schedule patient visits within protocol visit windows. This also minimizes the amount of missing visits for key data.

1.1.1 SDTMs and ADaMs Vitals

The first level is SDTMs and ADaMs vital checks, which are essential unit-level checks to assure SDTMs and ADaMs content are representative of raw data in standardized control terms and structure. In addition, dataset vitals and zero records checks assures correct data transfers as well as data requirements and assumptions.

The SDTMs and ADaMs mind maps show grouping of domains based on relationship to patients. SDTMs are grouped as Interventions, Trail Design, Special, Findings, Relationships and Events. For instance, checks on Findings domains, such as LB and QS, can use similar macro calls. Organizations can leverage this grouping with the types of checks performed. In Figure 1.2, key ADaMs from selected SDTMs are included in the mind map.

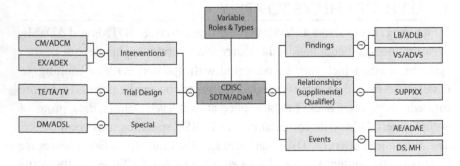

FIGURE 1.2   SDTMs and ADaMs mind map.

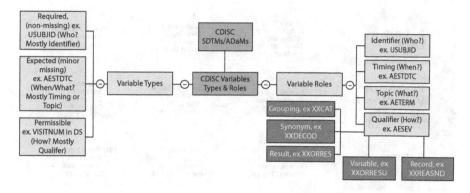

FIGURE 1.3   SDTM variable types and roles mind map.

SDTM Variable Types and Roles mind map shows multiple variable types and roles. This is useful to understand how and why data is mapped to variable types. In Figure 1.3, this mind map follows CDISC structure rules, which can be checked for compliance.

See Chapter 2 for examples of SDTMs and ADaMs vitals checks.

1.1.2 SDTMs and ADaM Data

The second level is SDTMs and ADaM data checks to assure higher data quality. Since adverse and lab data determine if patient safety is at risk and efficacy data determine how well patients are performing, there are many important checks at this level, including checks for duplicate records, data range and lab data. This verification process is often outlined in the data management plans of organizations.

When raw data is mapped and transferred to SDTMs and then to ADaMs, there should be no loss or change in data content or in analysis format. In Table 1.2, as data is transferred, checks assure each SDTM and ADaM variable is correctly populated to pass Pinnacle 21 check requirements.

The foundation of all checks in this book is based on the five channels of the CDISC Compliance Issues chart: Unit Level, Multiple

TABLE 1.2   Raw to SDTM to ADaMs Data Transfer

Data	Data Transfer Plan
Raw Data	Original data, horizontal structure, non-standard variable and values
SDTMs	XX and SUPPXX domains, vertical/normalized, standard variables and values
ADaMs	Analysis only from SAP, vertical/normalized, derived records

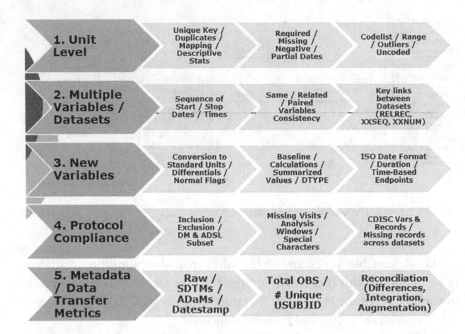

1. Unit Level	Unique Key / Duplicates / Mapping / Descriptive Stats	Required / Missing / Negative / Partial Dates	Codelist / Range / Outliers / Uncoded
2. Multiple Variables / Datasets	Sequence of Start / Stop Dates / Times	Same / Related / Paired Variables Consistency	Key links between Datasets (RELREC, XXSEQ, XXNUM)
3. New Variables	Conversion to Standard Units / Differentials / Normal Flags	Baseline / Calculations / Summarized Values / DTYPE	ISO Date Format / Duration / Time-Based Endpoints
4. Protocol Compliance	Inclusion / Exclusion / DM & ADSL Subset	Missing Visits / Analysis Windows / Special Characters	CDISC Vars & Records / Missing records across datasets
5. Metadata / Data Transfer Metrics	Raw / SDTMs / ADaMs / Datestamp	Total OBS / # Unique USUBJID	Reconciliation (Differences, Integration, Augmentation)

FIGURE 1.4   Five channels of CDISC compliance issues.

Variables/Datasets, New Variables, Protocol Compliance and Metadata/ Data Transfer Metrics. Many Pinnacle 21 checks can be summarized into these five channels. In Figure 1.4, each channel represents the breakdown of different sources of compliance issues. Within each channel, categories of checks are organized to apply check strategies. For example, the unit-level channel has subtopics such as unique keys, duplicates, mapping and descriptive stats as a subgroup and codelist, range, outliers and uncoded values in a second subgroup. These channels and categories identify and correct the source of the issue, such as a broken CDISC rule, a data or controlled terminology issue or a study design issue. In addition, these channels are consistent with Pinnacle 21 checks on controlled terminology compliance and SDTM structure consistency, format compliance, referential integrity and limits. Many of Pinnacle 21's common issues such as missing and issues with codelists, missing required variables, duplicate records and inconsistency between paired variables such as XXTEST/CD can be identified and corrected from these checks. The chapters explore each CDISC compliance channel.

Since the unit-level channel is one of the most important channels, essential dataset vital statistics assure no duplicate records or missing

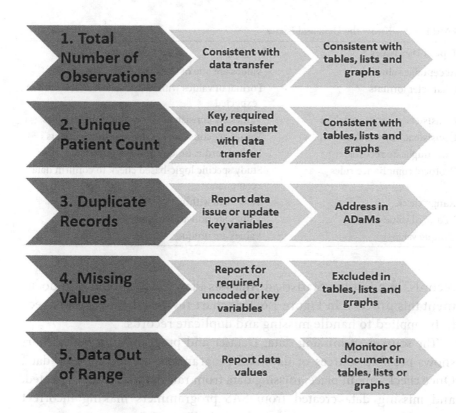

1. Total Number of Observations	Consistent with data transfer	Consistent with tables, lists and graphs
2. Unique Patient Count	Key, required and consistent with data transfer	Consistent with tables, lists and graphs
3. Duplicate Records	Report data issue or update key variables	Address in ADaMs
4. Missing Values	Report for required, uncoded or key variables	Excluded in tables, lists and graphs
5. Data Out of Range	Report data values	Monitor or document in tables, lists or graphs

FIGURE 1.5   Unit-level dataset vital stats.

required variables. In Figure 1.5, early dataset vital statistics checks are useful in rejecting incoming raw data. Other dataset vitals include total number of observations, unique patient count and data out of range.

Typically, in clinical data management departments, edit check programs identify data issues that do not meet protocol compliance. In Table 1.3, knowing the data and issues chart summarizes the types of issues that can impact data quality and inconsistency.

In clinical studies, when data issues from missing values in a required variable or duplicate records based on key variables exist, SAS program errors and warnings may occur since the programs do not expect them. This is because, in general, SAS programs assume data integrity to link related datasets together as well as meet data quality requirements to be meaningful. The non-missing, missing and dupli-cate records chart shows possible challenging LB cases when applying analysis windows. Often when these cases are found, clinical data man-agement needs to be queried to determine how best to address these

TABLE 1.3 Know the Data and Issues

Type of Data Issues	Brief Description
Acceptable values	Values are one of the valid values for variable
Character formats	Format of values within character variables are as expected
Consistency across variables	Values are consistent across multiple variables
Consistency across datasets	Values are consistent across multiple datasets
Non-duplicate records	Each record is unique and not duplicated
Protocol compliance rules	Study specific logic-based check to confirm data compliance
Range check	Values are within a specific range
Required value	Values are non-missing
Unique value	Values are unique

records. In addition, Statistical Analysis Plan (SAP) should also document this process. In Figure 1.6, this chart reviews the logic that needs to be applied to handle missing and duplicate records.

The sources of missing data: Dataset and programming issues chart shows possible sources of data and programmer-created missing data. Once checks are in place, missing data from raw datasets can be rejected, and missing data created from SAS programmers making incorrect assumptions can be corrected, as shown in Figure 1.7.

See Chapter 3 for examples of SDTMs and ADaMs data checks.

Challenges in assigning analysis visit windows in LB

By Group Variables	Date Exists?	Time Exists?	Value Exists?	Action
Non duplicate record	Y	Y	Y	Keep record
Duplicate records	Same	Same or Y/Missing Or Both Missing	Y/Y or Y/Missing	Take mean value and keep only one record
Duplicate records	Same	Not Same and Non-missing	Y/Y	Take most recent time record value
Duplicate records	Same	Missing	Y/Missing	Take non-missing value record
Duplicate records	Same	Missing	Missing	Keep only one record

FIGURE 1.6 Non-missing, missing and duplicate records.

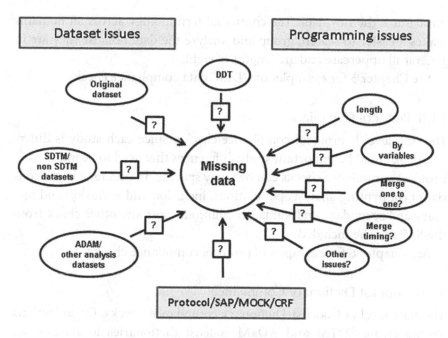

FIGURE 1.7   Sources of missing data: Dataset and programming issues.

1.1.3 CDISC Specifications Compliance

The third level is CDISC specifications compliance checks. CDISC speci-fication compliance checks confirm dataset rules are applied, such as vari-able and record sort order and the existence of key variables instead of data content checks, which are in other chapters. Strict dataset structure meta-data rules must be followed to standardize the process of raw data. Along with define.xml, this is an important submission package acceptance test to pass technical metadata requirements. If the submission package metadata cannot be properly loaded at the FDA, the FDA may reject the submission before it can review the actual data. The uniform structure of all domains makes it easier to search, group and analyze the data. In this book, SDTM IG 3.2 specifications are used.

See Chapter 4 for examples of CDISC specification compliance checks.

1.1.4 CDISC Data Compliance

The fourth level is CDISC data compliance check. CDISC data compliance checks confirm data rules are applied for each variable and multiple vari-able consistencies. Strict controlled terminology rules must be followed to standardize the raw data. The controlled terminology across all domains makes it easier to search, group and analyze the data because they are in general all uppercase and are lengths of eight.

See Chapter 5 for examples of CDISC data compliance checks.

1.1.5 Protocol Compliance

The fifth level is protocol compliance checks. Since each study is different, there could be important study differences that need to be monitored. Protocol compliance checks can be study specific. In general, checks consist of confirming analysis populations, inclusion and exclusion and primary and secondary endpoints. In addition, most any other check from the SAP may be included.

See Chapter 6 for examples of protocol compliance checks.

1.1.6 Codelist Dictionary Compliance

The final level is Codelist Dictionary compliance checks. Organizations should create SDTM and ADaM codelist dictionaries to confirm all unique values from categorical variables. One Excel file can be created with all SDTM codelists as columns in the same order as variables stored. This makes it easier to view and filter codelists across domains. Having an automated tool to refresh codelists keeps the codelist current with minimum effort. The alternative is to apply Proc FREQ on each categorical variable, which is very time consuming. Figure 1.8 shows how codelist names are generally the same as their corresponding variable names. Also, there should be consistency between codelists in DDT which are data definition tables or dataset specifications and SDTMs.

The second component to codelist dictionaries is to confirm SDTM codelists are consistent with the controlled terminology dictionary. Figure 1.9 shows the process of comparing and identifying inconsistencies in codelists. One Excel file can be created with values for SDTMs and controlled terminology dictionaries to flag differences with each other. With corrections to the SDTM codelists, the difference tool can be rechecked. Having an automated tool to review codelist differences keeps the codelist current with minimum effort. This is a very important step toward creating the define .xml file.

See Chapter 7 for examples of Codelist Dictionary compliance checks.

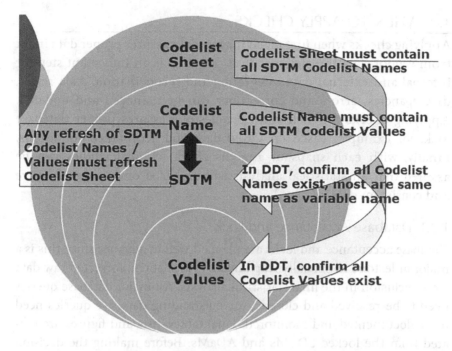

FIGURE 1.8   SDTM codelist: Names and values.

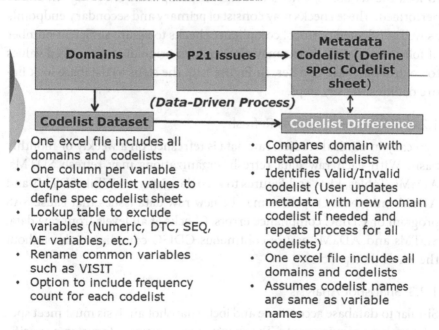

FIGURE 1.9   Define spec: Codelist dictionary/difference.

1.2 WHEN TO APPLY CHECKS

Applying checks when first receiving raw data assures proper data input from vendor data transfer specifications. This is an important step for internal and external data integration and reconciliation. As a result, discrepancies, errors and corrections can be managed and updated. Applying checks for each clinical milestone assures proper database lock, for example, based on QCed data and acceptance conditions. Finally, with each snapshot analysis check, clinical studies can be assured that all statistical analysis will be based on a comprehensive and consistent data.

1.2.1 Database Acceptance and Lock

Database acceptance and locks are planned well in advance since this is a major milestone to officially stop any new raw data or corrected raw data from inclusion in the final statistical analysis. All major database queries need to be resolved and closed. Any outstanding database queries need to be documented and monitored. Final tables, lists and figures are created from the locked SDTMs and ADaMs. Before making the decision to lock the database, extensive database acceptance checking should be performed. These checks may consist of primary and secondary endpoints as well as selected protocol compliance checks to assure sufficient number of follow-up visits. Checks may also confirm original and changed values to control database updates. In Figure 1.10, the steps to database lock figure outlines the key steps.

1.2.2 SDTMs and ADaMs Refresh

Typically in clinical studies, raw data is refreshed on a weekly or monthly basis. With each raw data refresh, organizations may refresh SDTMs, ADaMs, Tables, Lists and Figures to keep data in sync. While SDTMs and ADaMs may pass QC, there may be new raw data issues that cause SAS program or CDISC compliance errors. Checks at all levels from raw data, SDTMs and ADaMs assure continuous CDISC compliance throughout the whole data process.

1.2.3 Snapshot Analysis

Similar to database acceptance and lock, snapshot analysis must meet specific analysis requirements. The snapshot analysis may focus on a specific patient population or endpoint. Checks can be applied to assure correct snapshot analysis.

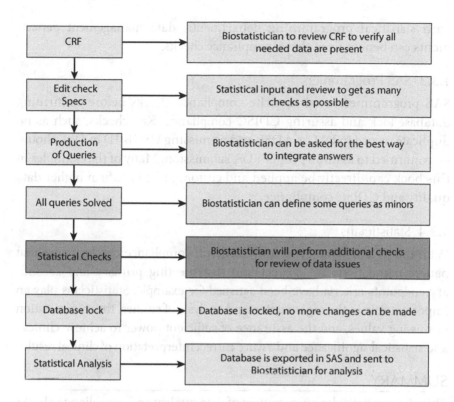

FIGURE 1.10   Steps to database lock.

1.3 CUSTOMIZED CHECKS FOR EACH CLIENT

When each department applies checks, different viewpoints of the data are confirmed to be consistent with expectations. This assures a unified story at the subject level. Example of these checks include site planning for scheduled patient visits, assuring site protocol compliance, database lock acceptance testing and primary and secondary endpoint checks.

1.3.1 Site Management

One of the standard planning tools from clinical data management to clinical sites is the scheduling of expected and missing patient follow-up visits. The site can then manage patient office visits to maintain protocol compliance. Meeting needs of clinical sites as well as continuous training on case report updates and controlled terminology improve data quality.

1.3.2 Data Management

The data management plan in many organizations details when and how checks are applied to assure protocol compliance and data quality. Along with statistical programming departments, data management departments can benefit from these compliance checks.

1.3.3 SAS Programmers

SAS programmers need to write compliance checks before confirming database lock and assuring CDISC compliance. Key checks, such as no duplicate record in DM or ADSL and no missing USUBJID in DM, should be confirmed to assure a proper FDA submission. Many of the examples in this book can directly be applied and customized to confirm higher data quality and CDISC compliance.

1.3.4 Statisticians

With the ADaMs One-Proc Away concept, compliance checks assure that patient populations are correct and that meeting primary and secondary endpoints criteria have been satisfied for example. Statisticians play an important role in the organization and analysis of studies, the minimization of missing values, and the assurance of sufficient power to achieve clinical, and statistical significance and assure correct interpretation of clinical results.

SUMMARY

This chapter provides an overview of data quality and compliance checks that are explained in each chapter. The unique approach of applying these checks assures everyone is on the same page to focus on data quality and CDISC compliance. By preparing with extensive CDISC rules, domain metadata and advanced SAS programming techniques, SAS programmers are able to control and correct compliance issues.

SAS Programming is an art that needs to be carefully constructed to facilitate ease of maintenance. Proper merging of datasets ensures correct linking of patient data as well as preventing artificial missing data. Having complete traceability of all patients from screening to end of study or lost to follow-up enables organizations to answer FDA questions as well as show complete control of the study. Finally, knowing how to take advantage of ADaM's One-Proc Away feature enables organizations to expedite the creation of summaries of both categorical and continue data. With proper documentation and understanding of where data and programming issues can occur, preventive measures can be taken to assure higher quality results; Topics presented in the appendix are Figure A.1 Anatomy of a SAS program, Figure A.2 Data model of datasets and key variables, Figure A.3 Subject disposition tree from enrollment to study completion and Table A.3 One-Proc Away Using Proc Tabulate: Knowing your Row and Column Options. This Proc Tabulate summary table is an overview of advanced options.

The SAS programming techniques applied in this book leverages the power of Proc SQL with macro creating, subqueries and multitasking features. Effective unit testing assures controlled steps are followed during the development progress. In addition, utilizing metadata is more intelligent programming, assuring higher quality results through automation and standardization. See in the appendix charts on Figure A.2 Data model of datasets and key variables, Figure A.4 Proc SQL joins mind map, Figure A.5 Proc SQL subqueries mind map, Table A.1 Four Key Metadata/ Dictionary Datasets, Table A.2 Proc SQL Productive Summary Sheet and Figure A.10 Effective unit testing concepts for Proc SQL.

Below is a list of useful dictionary dataset content from TABLES and COLUMNS used throughout the book.

- Dataset name

- Date of creation

- Number of observations and number of variables

- Whether the dataset is sorted, compressed, indexed

- Information for each variable

- Position (sequential number) in the dataset

  - Variable name

  - Type

  - Length

  - Format and informat

  - Label

Checking Excel files should be part of the compliance checking processing since many organizations use Excel files to store metadata. Excel files serve well to organize, store and update data that is controllable, manageable way and is easily accessible by SAS. In addition, SAS can create Excel files to communicate and exchange information, such as summary analysis or data issues. Multiple sheets can be created similar to Proc

PRINT of all datasets in a specific library for example. With Excel's data filter option, for example, anyone can search across multiple sheets, subset or group data very easily. In addition, additional columns can be added to keep track of any comments. Output Excel files can be used as input by statisticians to confirm complex calculations or by clinical data management, for example, to address data issues. In the appendix in Table A.8 are tips for processing Excel files, such as formulas to compare two columns and report if there is matching or not matching in the third column. In addition, there is a SAS utility to convert an Excel file with multiple sheets to multiple intermediate datasets.

Crosschecking tasks and issues with checklists assures all details are accounted for in a regulated environment. While these checklists are useful for QA, they can also be applied throughout the process of SDTM, ADaM and tables, lists and figure creation. In the appendix, are four checklists to guide organizations to CDISC compliant SDTMs and ADaMs that are error and warning-free Pinnacle 21 issues, which lead to creating define.xml from a define spec file. See in appendix – Table A.4 Raw Data to SDTMs to ADaMs Compliance Checklist, Table A.5 Clinical Study and CDISC Compliance Checklist, Table A.6 Pinnacle 21 Issues Checklist and Table A.7 Pinnacle 21 Define Spec to Define XML Checklist. The example macro names in the Raw Data to SDTMs to ADaMs Compliance Checklist are references only and are not included with the book. The macros represent the types of unit-level tasks needed to map and QC raw data to SDTMs and ADaMs.

CHAPTER 2

SDTMs and ADaMs Vital Checks

INTRODUCTION

SDTMs and ADaMs vital checks assure data integrity when data flows from raw data to SDTMs and then finally to ADaMs as shown in Figure 2.1. Dataset level checks include vitals, dataset transfer, group descriptive statistics, zero dataset records, and disposition population tree checks. Disposition population trees provide total accountability and traceability for all patients.

2.1 DATASET VITALS

Vital checks provide summarized information on key SDTMs and ADaMs so that organizations have the confidence to accept and process the data. Vital checks are also essential for database acceptance testing. The advantage of vital checks is that they can be customized for each SDTM and ADaM. Whether you are concerned about duplicate records or monitoring patient enrollment or deaths, for example, vital checks provide essential insights to your data without having to spend time digging into the details.

This example shows how to extract key vitals such as total number of records, patients, datetime stamps and duplicate records from ADSL. The COUNT() summary function, UNIQUE keyword, CASE block and subquery options were used in Proc SQL to summarize the results into one record. For each summarized result variable, a subquery with the appropriate conditions is applied. The CASE block and COUNT() function is used to identify duplicate records and is grouped by USUBJID.

1. Raw Data	2. Edit Check Process	3. Outcome
DM: Valid / Invalid Data VS: Valid / Invalid Data LB: Valid / Invalid Data AE: Valid / Invalid Data	a. Identify invalid data based on data management plan b. Isolate data issue c. Communicate findings to CDM	a. Monthly: Monitor improvements in invalid data b. Final: Use valid data in SDTMs, ADaMs, TLFs

FIGURE 2.1   Raw data flow.

Example 2.1.1: ADSL Vitals

```
proc sql;
create table dc as
select unique 'ADSL' as domain, "USUBJID" as keyvr_obs
    length=50
, count(USUBJID) as obs label="Total OBS"
, count(unique USUBJID) as ptc label="USUBJID count"
, b.ptc_saffl
, c.keygrpvr_dup, c.dc_dup
, d.dt_stamp
from adsl as a,
 (select count(unique USUBJID) as ptc_saffl label='USUBJID
    SAFFL count' from adsl where saffl='Y') as b,
(select unique compbl("USUBJID / USUBJID") as keygrpvr_dup
    label='Key Variables' length=50
 , case when count(USUBJID) = 1 then "No Duplicate Records "
   else 'Yes Duplicate Records' end as dc_dup label="duplicate
   records"
 from adsl group by USUBJID) as c,
(select unique input(scan(put(crdate, DATETIME16.), 1, ':'), date7.)
    format=date9. as dt_stamp label='Date Stamp' from sashelp.
    vtable
  where upcase(libname)="WORK" and upcase(memname)=upcase
  ("ADSL")) as d;
quit;
```

The results confirm no duplicate records in ADSL as well as the total number of patients, observations and datetime stamp. The results of each subquery create a new variable. In addition, the safety population PTC_SAFFL is displayed. The KEYVR_OBS and KEYGRPVR_DUP show USUBJID as the key variable.

Output

Obs	domain	keyvr_obs	obs	ptc	ptc_saffl	keygrpvr_dup	dc_dup	dt_stamp
1	ADSL	USUBJID	187	187	146	USUBJID / USUBJID	No Duplicate Records	01JAN2019

The next example is a more robust method to append vitals. With Proc SQL's OUTER UNION CORR, you can customize vitals with a list and count of all unique values from categorical variables or descriptive statistics on continuous variables instead of concatenating vitals. The difference in this method compared with the previous method is to create records instead of variables. The real power of each OUTER UNION CORR method is that additional summary information records can be created for any SDTM, ADaM, variable or condition.

Example 2.1.2: ADSL Vitals using OUTER UNION CORR

```
proc sql;
create table dc as
select unique "USUBJID" as adsl_vrs length=75
, count(USUBJID) as obs label="Total OBS"
, count(unique USUBJID) as num1 label="Record Count"
from adam.adsl as a

outer union corr
 select 'SAFFL' as adsl_vrs, count(unique USUBJID) as num1 from
    adam.adsl where saffl='Y'
outer union corr
 select unique compbl("USUBJID Duplicate Records") as adsl_vrs
 , case when count(USUBJID) = 1 then "No Duplicate Records "
 else "Yes Duplicate Records" end as char1
 from adam.adsl group by USUBJID
```

(Continued)

Example 2.1.2 (*Continued*): ADSL Vitals using OUTER UNION CORR

```
outer union corr
select 'ENRLDT (Min, Max)' as adsl_vrs, min(ENRLDT) as date1
   format=date9.,
max(ENRLDT) as date2 format=date9. from adam.
   adsl where ENRLDT > .

outer union corr
select unique 'ARM' as adsl_vrs, arm as char1,
count(USUBJID) as num1 from adam.adsl group by arm

outer union corr
select unique 'APHASE' as adsl_vrs, aphase as char1,
count(USUBJID) as num1 from adam.adsl group by aphase

outer union corr
select unique '101-006-003 Cohort/Enrollment Date' as adsl_vrs,
   aphase as char1,
count(USUBJID) as num1, ENRLDT as date1 from adam.adsl wh
   ere SUBJID='101-006-003';
quit;
```

DC displays ADSL's selected categorical variable unique values, counts and descriptive statistics. The first four records are similar to the previous method and records 5 to 13 display frequency counts of selected categorical variable values. This method allows for customization in the order of records and type of information to display from several SDTMs.

Output

Obs	adsl_vrs	obs	num1	char1	date1	date2
1	USUBJID	187	187		.	.
2	SAFFL	.	146		.	.
3	USUBJID Duplicate Records	.	.	No Duplicate Records	.	.
4	ENRLDT (Min, Max)	.	.		17APR2015	25SEP2017
5	ARM	.	146	■■■■■■	.	.
6	ARM	.	15	Not Assigned	.	.
7	ARM	.	26	Screen Failure	.	.
8	APHASE	.	11	Phase1	.	.
9	APHASE	.	21	Phase2	.	.
10	APHASE	.	81	Phase2 Cohort1	.	.
11	APHASE	.	32	Phase2 Cohort2	.	.
12	APHASE	.	42	Phase2 Cohort3	.	.
13	101-006-003 Cohort/Enrollment Date	.	1	Phase2 Cohort3	31OCT2016	.

Similar to Example 2.1.1, Example 2.1.3 extracts key vitals from ADAE. Since ADAE is multiple records per USUBJID, USUBJID and AESEQ are the key variables.

Example 2.1.3: ADAE Vitals

```
proc sql;
create table dc as
select unique 'ADAE' as domain, "USUBJID" as keyvr_obs
    length=50
, count(USUBJID) as obs label="Total OBS"
, count(unique USUBJID) as ptc label="USUBJID count"
, b.keygrpvr_dup, b.dc_dup
, c.dt_stamp
from adae as a,
 (select unique compbl("USUBJID / AESEQ") as keygrpvr_dup
    label='Key Variables' length=50
 , case when count(USUBJID) = 1 then "No Duplicate Records "
  else 'Yes Duplicate Records' end as dc_dup label="Duplicate
  records"
 from adae group by USUBJID, AESEQ) as b,
(select unique input(scan(put(crdate, DATETIME16.), 1, ':'), date7.)
    format=date9. as dt_stamp label='Date Stamp' from sashelp.
    vtable
  where upcase(libname)="WORK" and upcase (memname) =
    upcase ("ADAE")) as c;
quit;
```

DC confirms no duplicate records in ADAE as well as the total number of patients, observations and datetime stamp.

Output

Obs	domain	keyvr_obs	obs	ptc	keygrpvr_dup	dc_dup	dt_stamp
1	ADAE	USUBJID	100	4	USUBJID / AESEQ	No Duplicate Records	01JAN2019

As an alternative to Proc SQL for continuous variables, Proc MEANS can be used on ADTTE to extract N, MIN and MAX survival days by PARAMCD. The NWAY option forces only the highest level combination of all CLASS variables. The AUTONAME option uses the variable names as the root and appends as suffix, _N, _MIN and _MAX. The example below calculates the count, minimum and maximum survival days by PARAMCD, CNSR and EVNTDESC.

Example 2.1.4: ADTTE Vitals

```
proc means data=adam.adtte nway noprint maxdec=2;
class param paramcd cnsr evntdesc;
var aval;
output out=adtte1 (drop= _type_ _freq_) n= min= max=/
    autoname;
run;
```

The ADTTR1 output dataset can be viewed or merged back to the original dataset to include N, MIN and MAX survival times by PARAMCD. Partial results are displayed.

Output

EVNTDESC	AVAL_N	AVAL_Min
0 DEATH (AT ANY TIME) BEFORE DOCUMENTED PROGRESSION	2	184
PROGRESSION PER CHESON 2007 AT A SCHEDULED ASSESSMENT OR IN BETWEEN SCHEDULED ASSESSMENTS AND AFTER		
0 ASCT	1	252

To assure consistency across domains, it is important to confirm patient counts. The next example compares patient counts across EX, DS, LB and AE. This check confirms greater than or equal patient counts from the first to the last SDTM listed. In general, this check should be applied as IE >= DM >= EX and DM >= DV, AE, DS. The IE domain is expected to have the highest patient count over other domains since screen failures are included in IE.

Example 2.1.5: SDTM Core Checks

```
* SDTM patient counts checks: IE >= DM >= EX, DM >= DV/AE/DS;
proc sql;
create table dc as
select unique "USUBJID" as keyvr_obs length=50
, count(unique USUBJID) as dm_ptc label="USUBJID count"
, b.ex_ptc, c.ds_ptc, d.lb_ptc, e.ae_ptc
from dm as a,
(select count (unique USUBJID) as EX_PTC label='USUBJID
    count' from ex) as b,
(select count (unique USUBJID) as DS_PTC label='USUBJID
    count' from ds) as c,
(select count (unique USUBJID) as LB_PTC label='USUBJID
    count' from lb) as d,
(select count (unique USUBJID) as AE_PTC label='USUBJID
    count' from ae) as e;
quit;
```

The results show patient counts across DM, EX, DS, LB and AE. We see that DM has the largest number of patients as expected with equal number in DS followed by smaller patient counts in LB and AE. In this example, a flag can be created to identify any incorrect order of patient counts.

Output

			Page Break			
Obs	keyvr_obs	dm_ptc	EX_PTC	DS_PTC	LB_PTC	AE_PTC
1	USUBJID	187	150	187	2	4

2.2 DATA TRANSFERS

Since data is constantly transferred from vendors with different schedules based on the type of data, organizations must be proactive in controlling the acceptance of each data transfer. With each data transfer, organizations must be confident that all data received is correct by confirming database values equal SAS dataset values. Often, truncation can occur due to faulty coding or values being set to missing when SAS did not understand the conversion due to date storage formats.

The examples in this section are essential clinical data metadata for effective data transfers. The dictionary datasets, TABLES and COLUMNS contain much of this information and can easily be accessed. See Table A.1 Four Key Metadata/Dictionary Datasets in the appendix for more details. Any metadata information outside of TABLES and COLUMNS datasets can be created as customized checks using SAS.

Below are examples of custom metadata that can be created from Proc SQL:

- Confirm required files, datasets and variables

- Confirm total number of datasets and datetime stamps

- Confirm total number of observations and patients

- Confirm total number and type of variables and attributes

- Confirm required non-missing variables

- Confirm no duplicate records

- Confirm order of variables

- Confirm new variable lengths are not less than maximum variable lengths

- Confirm complete codelist dictionary, ex. lab units

- Monitor descriptive statistics on key categorical and continuous variables

- Compare and contrast previous datasets and attributes to monitor increase or decrease in datasets, records or variables

The SAS examples below extract metadata from each data transfer without having to hard code the name of each domain. In addition with SAS, code can be written to email data transfer summaries to teams for monitoring. While most data transfers are expected to be a complete replacement of the previous version, some data transfers may include only new or changed data. This may require special handling to append to the old data or replace original values.

The Proc SQL example below confirms correct patient counts and creation dates for the three oncology SDTM domains – TU, TR and RS. In general, it is expected that these domains should have similar patient counts and creation dates. This example can be modified to cross-check consistency for any combination of raw, SDTMs and ADaMs. Patient counts and datetime stamp subqueries are created for each domain.

Example 2.2.1: Data Transfer

```
proc sql;
create table dc as
select unique
count(unique USUBJID) as tu_ptc label="USUBJID count"
, b.*, c.*, d.*, e.*, f.*, g.*
from sdtm.tu as a,
(select count(unique USUBJID) as tr_ptc from sdtm.tr) as b,
(select count(unique USUBJID) as rs_pct from sdtm.rs) as c,
(select count(unique USUBJID) as tu_tr_rs_pct from tu_tr_rs) as d,
(select unique input(scan(put(crdate, DATETIME16.), 1, ':'), date7.)
    format=date9. as tu_stamp from sashelp.vtable
  where upcase(libname)="SDTM" and upcase(memname)=
    upcase("TU")) as e,
(select unique input(scan(put(crdate, DATETIME16.), 1, ':'), date7.)
    format=date9. as tr_stamp from sashelp.vtable
  where upcase(libname)="SDTM" and upcase(memname)=
    upcase("TR")) as f,
(select unique input(scan(put(crdate, DATETIME16.), 1, ':'), date7.)
    format=date9. as rs_stamp from sashelp.vtable
  where upcase(libname)="SDTM" and upcase(memname)=
    upcase("RS")) as g;
quit;
```

The results show expected patient counts and creation date for each oncology domain. Big differences in data timestamps for TR and RS could indicate that RS needs to be refreshed. The TR_TU_RS_PCT patient count is from the combined dataset form TU, TR and RS, which is from another example.

Output

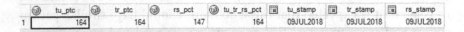

	tu_ptc		tr_ptc		rs_pct		tu_tr_rs_pct		tu_stamp		tr_stamp		rs_stamp
1	164		164		147		164		09JUL2018		09JUL2018		09JUL2018

Another type of transfer check can be applied to SAS programs to confirm correct sequence of source and QC program and log date stamps. In general, any SAS program updated is followed by rerunning the SAS program. In addition, the corresponding QC program is updated and rerun. This sequence of datetime stamps assures QC programs always follow source program logs. The SAS macro below first creates four datasets to store the program names and datetime stamps of all source and QC programs and then compare their datetime stamps by program name. The FILENAME statement references each SAS program path name. Dataset functions are used to open datasets, count number of records and read files, as well as get metadata information. From this check, organizations can quickly identify if any SAS source or QC program must be rerun or if any source or QC program is missing. Note that this QA check is robust to process any number of SAS programs and log files because the program is generated using metadata instead of manually hardcoding each SAS program name. The one macro is called four times, one for each type of SAS file, source program, log, QC program and log. Once the intermediate datasets are created, they are joined and then compared for any incorrect sequence order. Proc SQL's FULL JOIN links by the root SAS program name and keeps records from all datasets. In addition, the COALESCE() function assures the FILE_ NAME variable is not missing.

Example 2.2.2: File Datetime Stamp Checks

```
%macro dstamp(dsnme=, pathdir=, ext=sas);
* SAS program and log path names;
filename dirRef "&pathdir";

data &dsnme (where =(index(file_name, ".&ext") > 0));
dirID=dopen("dirRef");
num_of_files=dnum(dirID);
```

(Continued)

Example 2.2.2 (*Continued*): File Datetime Stamp Checks

```
&dsnme._path="&pathdir";
keep &dsnme._path file_name file_name2 &dsnme._dt;
format &dsnme._dt datetime16. file_name2 $50.;

* Loop through each file;
do i=1 to num_of_files;
 file_name=dread(dirID, i);
 rc1=filename("fRef",catx("/","&pathdir", file_name));
 fid=fopen("fRef");

 if fid > 0 then do;
  full_name=finfo(fid, "FileName");
  bytes=finfo(fid, "File Size (bytes)");
  &dsnme._dt=input(finfo(fid, "Last Modified"), anydtdtm.);
  owner=finfo(fid, "Owner Name");
  rc2=fclose(fid);
   * remove extentions;
  file_name2 = tranwrd(strip(file_name), '.sas', '');
  file_name2 = tranwrd(strip(file_name2), '.log', '');
  output;
 end;
end;
 fId = fClose( fId );
run;
%mend dstamp;
%dstamp(dsnme=s_sas, pathdir=\\analysis\program\tfl);
%dstamp(dsnme=s_log, pathdir=\\analysis\program\tfl, ext=log);
%dstamp(dsnme=q_sas, pathdir=\\analysis\validation\tfl);
%dstamp(dsnme=q_log, pathdir=\\analysis\validation\tfl, ext=log);

* Combine and create issues flag;
* xx.sas and v_xx.sas program names are combined;
proc sql;
create table b_dstamp as
 select unique coalesce(ss.file_name2, qs.file_name2) as file_name,
 s_sas_dt, q_sas_dt, s_log_dt, q_log_dt
```

(*Continued*)

Example 2.2.2 (*Continued*): File Datetime Stamp Checks

```
, case when s_log_dt > q_log_dt then 'Source log is after QC
    log' else ' ' end as issue
  from s_sas as ss full join q_sas as qs on ss.file_name2 =
    substr(qs.file_name2, 3)
  full join s_log as sl on ss.file_name2 = sl.file_name2
  full join q_log as ql on ss.file_name2 = substr(ql.file_name2, 3);
quit;

proc print data=b_dstamp noobs;
  where file_name > '' and nmiss(s_sas_dt, q_sas_dt, s_log_dt,
    q_log_dt)=0;
run;
```

The sample output below shows for each file name, the source, QC SAS program and log datetime stamps. In addition, the last column, ISSUES, displays a message if files are out of sequence, or if the source SAS program date is after the log date. Out of sequence dates necessitate a rerun of the SAS and QC programs. Missing values in the datetime stamp columns indicate that either the source or QC SAS program or SAS log file is missing. This information can help manage resources and gaps in tasks. Along with scanning each source and QC SAS log, this is a great QA tool to perform for any snapshot analysis or FDA submission. In general, the convention prefix is T_ for tables, L_ for lists and F_ for figures.

Output

file_name	s_sas_dt	q_sas_dt	s_log_dt	q_log_dt	issue
f_dor_crprc3	01JUN18:10:54:10	01JUN18:11:02:04	10JUL18:12:26:49	10JUL18:12:47:47	
f_dorc3	13JUL18:17:22:04	01JUN18:11:01:13	13JUL18:17:22:52	13JUL18:17:23:09	
f_forest_cr_addcov	20JUN18:11:03:27	18JUN18:10:50:28	23JUL18:09:13:54	23JUL18:09:19:45	
f_forest_cr_keyc3	06JUL18:07:10:55	05JUL18:14:13:55	10JUL18:12:02:53	10JUL18:12:49:44	
f_forest_crc3	06JUL18:07:01:26	05JUL18:14:08:26	10JUL18:12:02:48	10JUL18:12:49:42	

The next example provides automatic comparison between SDTMs from one library with similar SDTMs in a second library. In this example, Proc SQL accesses the VCOLUMN dataset from the WORK library and CLASS dataset to create DS_DIFF. For testing purpose, the CLASS dataset is created. The second DATA step will then loop through each record in DS_DIFF to create Proc COMPARE code for CLASS. The condition for MEMNAME can be updated to include all SDTMs. This same process can loop through each SDTM in a library without having to hard code each SDTM name. CALL EXECUTE contains the Proc COMPARE syntax, which compares the same SDTMs from two different libraries. Other Proc COMPARE options such as NOVALUES WARNING NOPRINT converts dataset differences into warnings in SAS logs, which make it easier to identify.

Example 2.2.3: Automatically Compare Old and Updated SDTMs

```
data class;
name = 'Alfred';
age=14;
sex='F';
height=75;
weight=100;
run;

proc sql;
create table ds_diff as
select unique memname
from sashelp.vcolumn where upcase(libname)='WORK' and
    upcase(memname) = 'CLASS';
quit;

data ds_diff1;
set ds_diff;

memname_ot = strip('std' || strip(put(_n_, 3.)));
call execute('proc compare data=work.'
|| memname
|| ' compare= sashelp.' || memname || ' listall out= ' || memname_ot
    || ' outnoequal; run;' );
run;
```

The first screenshot shows the SAS generated Proc COMPARE syntax for CLASS from the CALL EXECUTE statement. The second screenshot shows the partial results of Proc COMPARE. As expected, there are differences between the two CLASS datasets.

Output

```
NOTE: CALL EXECUTE generated line.
1          + proc compare data=work.CLASS                              compare= sashelp.CLASS
std1   outnoequal; run;

NOTE: There were 1 observations read from the data set WORK.CLASS.
NOTE: There were 19 observations read from the data set SASHELP.CLASS.
NOTE: The data set WORK.STD1 has 1 observations and 7 variables.
NOTE: PROCEDURE COMPARE used (Total process time):
      real time            0.01 seconds
      cpu time             0.00 seconds
```

```
                    Variables with Unequal Values

          Variable  Type  Len1 Len2  Ndif    MaxDif


          sex       CHAR    1    1     1
          height    NUM     8    8     1      6.000
          weight    NUM     8    8     1     12.500
```

-------------------------------- Page Break --------------------------------

```
                    The COMPARE Procedure
        Comparison of WORK.CLASS with SASHELP.CLASS
                       (Method=EXACT)


          Value Comparison Results for Variables
```

Obs	||	Base Value sex	Compare Value Sex
	||	_	_
	||		
1	||	F	M

2.3 GROUP DESCRIPTIVE STATISTICS

This section introduces a new method to quickly add group descriptive statistics to any dataset. With this innovative technique, many expansions such as adding summary information at the detail level is possible. Many of the examples in this book utilize this SAS programming technique. The examples below show how easy it is to add descriptive statistics including MIN, MAX, MEAN and Q1 to your datasets. The first example stores MIN and MAX values of AGE into one variable. Without a GROUP BY clause, Proc SQL performs an overall summary.

Example 2.3.1: Group Descriptive Statistics Checks by Overall

```
proc sql;
create table dc as
select unique 'ADSL' as domain,
  compbl("SUBJECTID / AGE") as key_grp_vr length=50
  , catx(' ', 'Min=', put(min(age), best.), ', Max=', put(max(age),
    best.)) as dc_rslt label="Data Check Results For:" length=50
  from adsl;
quit;
```

The results show group descriptive statistics for ADSL AGE. This method can be applied to monitor descriptive statistics for any raw, SDTM or ADaM.

Output

Obs	domain	key_grp_vr	dc_rslt
1	ADSL	SUBJECTID / AGE	Min= 21 , Max= 76

The second example has separate subqueries for each summary descriptive statistics. This method allows more flexibility to summarize based on any condition, any variable or any descriptive statistics instead of just one variable for overall statistics.

Example 2.3.2: Group Descriptive Statistics Checks Using Subqueries

```
proc sql;
create table dc as
select unique 'ADPCR' as domain, "USUBJID" as keyvr_obs
    length=50
, count(unique USUBJID) as ptc label="USUBJID count"
, b.n_peak, b.mean_peak, b.min_peak, b.max_peak
from adpcrs (where=(aphasen in (2.1, 2.2))) as a
```

(Continued)

Example 2.3.2 (*Continued*): Group Descriptive Statistics Checks Using Subqueries

```
, (select unique count(unique USUBJID) as n_peak, mean(peakval)
    as mean_peak format=best., min(peakval) as min_peak
    format=best., max(peakval) as max_peak format=best. from adpcrs
    where peakval > . and paramcd='nCART' and aphasen in (2.1,
    2.2)) as b;
quit;
```

The results show group descriptive statistics for peak count, mean, min and max peaks for ADPCR.PEAK.

Output

Obs	domain	keyvr_obs	ptc	n_peak	mean_peak	min_peak	max_peak
1	ADPCR	USUBJID	3	3	575.14641333	48.80304	1513.6922

The third example uses GROUP BY LBTESTCD to display descriptive statistics by LBTESTCD. This method is useful for by-group processing and can be repeated for LBSTNRLO, LBSTNRHI and LBSTRESN. This is an alternative method to Proc MEANs with BY statement.

Example 2.3.3: Group Descriptive Statistics Checks Using GROUP BY

```
PROC SQL;
create table dc as
select distinct domain, lbtestcd, lbornrlo, lbornrhi, min(lborres)
    as lborres_minval, max(lborres) as lborres_maxval
from lb group by lbtestcd;
quit;
```

The results show group descriptive statistics for MIN and MAX values for LB BCELL.

Output

Obs	DOMAIN	LBTESTCD	LBORNRLO	LBORNRHI	lborres_minval	lborres_maxval
1	LB	BCELL			0.050866281	BLQ

The final example uses Proc MEANS to extract descriptive statistics on AGE and then join the dataset back to the original dataset.

Example 2.3.4: Group Descriptive Statistics Checks using Proc MEANS

```
proc means data=adsl noprint;
var age;
where saffl = "Y" and aphasen in (2.1, 2.2);
output out=dca (drop= _type_ _freq_) q1=age_q1 min=age_min
    median=age_med q3=age_q3 max=age_max;
run;

proc sql;
create table dcb as
 select a.*, b.* from adsl as a, dca as b;
quit;
```

The partial results show AGE group descriptive statistics merged back to each record in the original dataset.

Output

Obs	age_q1	age_min	age_med	age_q3	age_max
1	51	23	58	64	76

FPDDT2C	PSURVFL	PDTHFL	age_q1	age_min	age_med	age_q3	age_max
			51	23	58	64	76
			51	23	58	64	76

2.4 ZERO DATASET RECORDS

While we generally do not expect datasets with zero records, sometimes errors happen in raw data transfer or SAS programs, which cause zero records in datasets. The Proc SQL examples below show several methods to confirm no zero records issue in SDTMs or ADaMs. DC1 stores any SDTMs or ADaM with zero records. DC2 stores the number of records for each SDTM and ADaM.

Example 2.4.1: Dataset Records Count Check

```
proc sql;
  create table dc1 as
  select libname, memname, nobs from dictionary.tables where
    libname in ('SDTM' 'ADAM') and nobs eq 0;
  create table dc2 as
  select libname, memname, nobs from dictionary.tables where
    libname inv ('SDTM' 'ADAM') order by nobs;
quit;
```

The results for DC2 dataset are useful to monitor the total number of records in each domain.

Output

Obs	libname	memname	nobs
1	SDTM	SUPPDD	6
2	SDTM	TA	14
3	SDTM	TE	14
4	SDTM	SUPPMO	17
5	SDTM	SUPPSS	21

In this example, a test XX dataset is created with zero records. The DC dataset is created to indicate a PASS or FAILed check for zero records, which means that there was at least one dataset with zero records. Notice that libnames SDTM and ADAM need to be predefined.

Example 2.4.2: Zero Dataset Records Check

```
* Condition test to show zero records check works for WORK
   directory;
proc sql;
create table xx like sashelp.class;
run;

proc sql;
create table dc as
select unique libname, memname, nobs
, case when nobs = 0 then 'FAIL: Zero Records'
else 'PASS: Records Exist' end as dc_rslt label="Data Check
   Results For:" length=75
from dictionary.tables where libname in ('SDTM' 'ADAM' 'WORK');
quit;
```

The results are useful to confirm if any zero records in datasets. XX dataset has zero records.

Output

WORK	XX	0	FAIL: Zero Records

2.5 DISPOSITION POPULATION TREES (SAFFL, ITTFL)

Creating and monitoring disposition population trees keep track of patients as they enter the study, complete schedule visits and then exit the study. While a number of patients may complete the study, there are many scenarios. Some patients may be terminated or withdraw. Some patients can experience serious adverse events, which can result in death. In addition, some patients may be lost to follow-up. Proc TABULATE is ideal to display a hierarchy of categories as well as relationships between patient populations. The first table is a hierarchy of rows (population flags) and columns (treatment group), and the second table is nested so that you see the counts based on all possible combinations of population flags- SAFFFL, MITT and treatment groups.

Example 2.5.1: Disposition Population Trees Check

```
title 'ADSL: Populations, SAFFFL, MITT';
proc tabulate data=ADSL missing noseps;
class saffl mittfl trt01p;
tables (saffl all mittfl all) , (trt01p all)*(n='N' COLPCTN='%'*f=5.1);
run;

title 'ADSL: Nested, SAFFFL, MITT';
proc tabulate data=ADSL missing noseps;
class saffl mittfl trt01p;
tables (trt01p*saffl*mittfl all)*(n='');
run;
```

From the table below, rows represent the different population flag values and the columns represent the different treatment group assignments. With Proc TABULATE, disposition tables can be displayed as hierarchy as in the first table or nested as in the second table.

Output

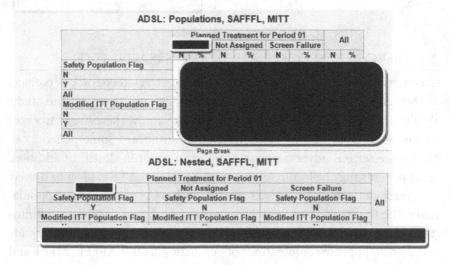

2.6 SDTM ONCOLOGY DOMAIN

For oncology studies, additional SDTMs required are TU for tumor identi-fication, TR for tumor measurements and RS for tumor results. An impor-tant integrity check is to confirm these three SDTM links are not broken since tumors can split, merge or disappear. Both identification and date variables need to be in sync so that a single oncology domain can be cre-ated to get an overall big picture across measurements and results. Once a single dataset from TU, TR and RS is created, a comprehensive review of the patient's data with all raw data measurements and evaluations can be more easily performed.

The Proc SQL example below links TU, TR and RS. The left join assures all TU records are kept as the master list. As an alternative, a FULL JOIN can be applied to identify any extra patient records from TR or RS. For one record per patient, identification variables are linked and for many to many records per patients, date variables are also linked. See example in data transfer check section below to confirm correct data transfer based on number of unique patients and creation dates.

Example 2.6.1: SDTM Oncology Domain Check

```
proc sql;
  create table tu_tr_rs as
  select tu.*, tr.*, rs.*
  from sdtm.tu as tu
  left join  sdtm.tr as tr on tu.usubjid = tr.usubjid and tu.TULNKID
    = tr.TrLNKID and tu.tudtc = tr.trdtc
  left join  sdtm.rs as rs on tr.usubjid = rs.usubjid and tr.trdtc =
    rs.rsdtc;
quit;
```

SUMMARY

This chapter provides examples of SDTMs and ADaMs vital checks. At a high level, core and group descriptive checks provide quick information on the integrity of the data. Whether it is raw, SDTMs or ADaMs, dataset level checks must always be applied with each refresh of the raw data. In addition, as more new CDISC rules are defined, additional steps should be taken to confirm these new and more complicated rules. In additional to the traditional data management steps to check the quality of data, the CDISC compliance checks in this publication will expedite FDA's review in an automated and standardized process.

CHAPTER 3

SDTMs and ADaMs Data Checks

INTRODUCTION

SDTMs and ADaMs data checks are the heart of the five channels of CDISC compliance issues chart in Figure 1.4, which assures higher data quality. Since all raw data is now standardized to controlled terms, there are many opportunities for cross-checking data. There are many examples in this chapter to identify and manage each type of check. In addition, multiple variable dependencies can be confirmed and corrected. Many of these data-level checks are also applicable to ADaMs. The SDTMs and ADaM data-level checks are consistent with Pinnacle 21 checks.

3.1 DUPLICATE RECORDS

Checking to confirm duplicate records do not exist is critical for each domain. Domains should be either one record per subject or multiple records per subject. For those domains that are multiple records per subject, it is important to check for duplicate records based on all key variables and on XXSEQ variable. The examples in this section can be applied on any domain after key variables have been identified. Below is an example of an AE domain.

In general, AE has these key variables: USUBJID, AESTDTC, AEENDTC, AETERM, AESEV, AESER.

	STUDYID	DOMAIN	USUBJID	AESEQ	AETERM	AEMODIFY	AEDECOD	AEBODSYS	AESEV	AESER	AEACN	AEREL	AESTDTC
1	CDISC01	AE	CDISC01.1000.	1	AGITATED	AGITATION	Agitation	Psychiatric dis..	MILD	N	DOSE NOT C.	POSSIBLY RE..	2003-05
2	CDISC01	AE	CDISC01.1000.	2	ANXIETY		Anxiety	Psychiatric dis..	MODERATE	N	DOSE NOT C.	POSSIBLY RE..	2003-05
3	CDISC01	AE	CDISC01.1000.	3	DECREASED.		Decreased app..	Metabolism an..	MILD	N	DOSE NOT C.	POSSIBLY RE..	2003-08
4	CDISC01	AE	CDISC01.1000.	1	DIARRHEA		Diarrhoea	Gastrointestina..	MILD	N	DOSE NOT C.	NOT RELATED	2004-01
5	CDISC01	AE	CDISC01.1000.	2	HEMORRHOI.		Haemorrhoids	Gastrointestina..	MODERATE	N	DOSE NOT C.	NOT RELATED	2004-01
6	CDISC01	AE	CDISC01.1000.	3	HEADACHE		Headache	Nervous syste..	MILD	N	DOSE NOT C.	NOT RELATED	2004-01
7	CDISC01	AE	CDISC01.1000.	4	VOMIT	VOMITING	Vomiting	Gastrointestina..	MODERATE	N	DRUG INTER..	POSSIBLY RE..	2004-02
8	CDISC01	AE	CDISC01.1000.	5	VOMIT	VOMITING	Vomiting	Gastrointestina..	SEVERE	Y	DRUG INTER..	POSSIBLY RE..	2004-02
9	CDISC01	AE	CDISC01.2000.	1	ANXIETY		Anxiety	Psychiatric dis..	SEVERE	N	DOSE NOT C.	POSSIBLY RE..	2003-10
10	CDISC01	AE	CDISC01.2000.	2	NAUSEA INTE.		Nausea	Gastrointestina..	SEVERE	N	DOSE NOT C.	POSSIBLY RE..	2003-10
11	CDISC01	AE	CDISC01.2000.	3	CONSTIPATIO.		Constipation	Gastrointestina..	MODERATE	N	DOSE NOT C.	NOT RELATED	2003-12
12	CDISC01	AE	CDISC01.2000.	4	TIREDNESS		Fatigue	General disord..	SEVERE	N	DOSE NOT C.	POSSIBLY RE..	2003-12
13	CDISC01	AE	CDISC01.2000.	5	LEFT KNEE P.		Arthralgia	Musculoskelet..	MILD	N	DRUG WITHD..	NOT RELATED	2004-02
14	CDISC01	AE	CDISC01.2000.	1	MUSCLE SPA..		Muscle spasms	Musculoskelet..	MILD	N	DOSE NOT C.	NOT RELATED	2004-01
15	CDISC01	AE	CDISC01.2000.	2	PALPITATION.		Palpitations	Cardiac disord..	MILD	N	DOSE NOT C.	NOT RELATED	2004-01
16	CDISC01	AE	CDISC01.2000.	3	LIGHTHEADE.		Dizziness	Nervous syste..	MILD	N	DOSE NOT C.	NOT RELATED	2004-02

The data check below confirms that USUBJID, AESTDTC, AEENDTC, AETERM, AESEV and AESER are unique (Summary Level).

The Proc SQL example below creates DC_AE1 dataset. This code includes a variable to document the key variables, logic to apply grouping by key variables and the count of USUBJID to identify duplicate records. The KEY_GRP_VR is a combination of the key variables. The CASE block has the logic with the summary function COUNT(). Note that without the GROUP BY clause, the summary function will be based on all records instead of the key variables.

Example 3.1.1: Duplicate Records Check by Key Variables

```
proc sql;
create table dc_ae1 as
select unique
  compbl("usubjid / aestdtc, aeendtc, aeterm, aesev, aeser") as
    key_grp_vr length=50
, case when count(usubjid) = 1 then 'PASS; Duplicate Records
  do Not Exist'
else 'FAIL; Duplicate Records Exist' end as ae_dup label="Work:
  AE duplicate
records" lengt=75 from work.ae group by usubjid, aestdtc,
  aeendtc, aeterm, aesev, aeser; quit;
```

This data check below shows no duplicate records by USUBJID, AESTDTC, AEENDTC, AETERM, AESEV or AESER. The KEY_GRP_VR variable documents which key variables were used to check for duplicate records.

Output

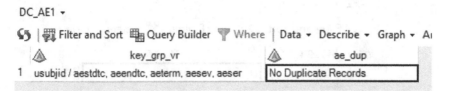

The next data check example confirms USUBJID and AESEQ are unique (Summary Level).

Since AESEQ is created as a record counter for each USUBJID and is based on key variables, it is best practice to confirm USUBJID and AESEQ do not have duplicate records. The KEY_GRP_VR is a combination of USUBID and AESEQ. The CASE block has the logic with the summary function COUNT(). Note that without the GROUP BY clause, the summary function will be based on all records instead of the key variables.

Example 3.1.2: Duplicate Records by AESEQ at Summary Level

```
proc sql;
create table dc_ae2 as
select unique
  compbl("usubjid / aeseq") as key_grp_vr length=50
  , case when count(usubjid) = 1 then 'PASS: Duplicate Records
    do Not Exist'
  else 'FAIL: Duplicate Records Exist' end as ae_dup label="Work:
    AE duplicate
records" length=75 from work.ae group by usubjid, aeseq; quit;
```

This data check shows no duplicate records by USUBJID, AESEQ. The KEY_GRP_VR variable documents which key variables were used to check for duplicate records.

Output

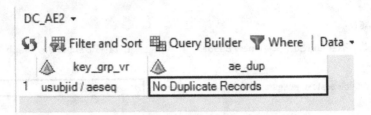

The next data check example confirms USUBJID and AESEQ are unique (Detail Level).

Since AESEQ is created as a record counter for each USUBJID and is based on key variables, it is best practice to confirm USUBJID and AESEQ do not have duplicate records. The DUPCNT variable is added to AE. Any DUPCNT > 1 indicates duplicate records.

Example 3.1.3: Duplicate Records by AESEQ at Detail Level

```
proc sql;
create table dc as
  create table dc as
  select a.*, b.dupcnt
  from work.ae as a  left join
    (select usubjid, aeseq, count(usubjid) as dupcnt label='Duplicate
    record count' from work.ae group by usubjid, aeseq)
  ) as b on a.usubjid=b.usubjid and a.aeseq=b.aeseq;
quit;
```

Output

AETOXGR	AESTDTC	AEENDTC	AESTDY	AEENDY	AEENRTPT	AEENTPT	dupcnt
2	2018-05-14	2018-05-14		.	BEFORE	END OF STUDY	1
1	2018-05-11	2018-05-11		.	BEFORE	END OF STUDY	1
1	2018-05-08	2018-05-08		.	BEFORE	END OF STUDY	1
3	2018-04-14	2018-04-25		.	BEFORE	END OF STUDY	1
1	2018-05-01	2018-05-01		.	BEFORE	END OF STUDY	1

3.2 MISSING VALUES IN REQUIRED VARIABLES

Missing values in required variables can cause SAS program errors as well as prevent raw data to SDTM refreshes. To prevent these issues, organizations should be proactive to confirm non-missing required variables. The example below shows ASTDT, AGE and AECECOD PASSed the non-missing required check, but the AENDT FAILed the non-missing required check. The Proc SQL code in this example is useful to identify if at least one record has a missing value by using the NMISS() summary function. The last two examples show two methods to check for non-missing required variable using function NMISS() and $CTNMISS format. Note that function NMISS() also works on character variables even though it is a numeric function. The $CTNMISS format converts all non-missing character values to 1 so that it's easier to identify. The NMISS format is similar but for numeric variables. Note that partial dates in AESTDTC could lead to missing ASTDT. In addition, at the ADaM level, ASTDT may be imputed, so missing ASTDT may indicate impute issue. This check can be repeated for USUBJID, AEREL, AESEV, AETERM, EXTRT, EPOCH and SUPPAE.AETRTEM and primary and secondary endpoints.

Example 3.2.1: Missing Values in Required Variable

```
* ADAE.ASTDT;
proc sql;
create table dc as
select unique 'ADAE' as domain,
  compbl("SUBJECTID / ASTDT") as key_grp_vr length=50
, case when nmiss(ASTDT) >= 1 then 'FAIL: Required Variable
    has at least one Missing Value'
  else 'PASS: Required Variable Does Not have any Missing
    Values' end as dc_rslt label="Data Check Results For:" length=200
  from adae;
quit;

* ADAE.AENDT;
proc sql;
create table dc as
select unique 'ADAE' as domain,
  compbl("SUBJECTID / AENDT") as key_grp_vr length=50
```

(Continued)

Example 3.2.1 (*Continued*): Missing Values in Required Variable

```
, case when nmiss(AENDT) >= 1 then 'FAIL: Required Variable
    has at least one Missing Values'
  else 'PASS: Required Variable Does Not have any Missing
     Values' end as dc_rslt label="Data Check Results For:" length=75
 from adae;
quit;
* ADSL.AGE;
proc sql;
create table dc as
select unique 'ADSL' as domain,
  compbl("SUBJECTID / AGE") as key_grp_vr length=50
 , case when nmiss(AGE) >= 1 then 'FAIL: Required Variable has
    at least one Missing Values'
  else 'PASS: Required Variable Does Not have any Missing
     Values' end as dc_rslt label="Data Check Results For:" length=75
   from adsl;
quit;

* ADAE.AEDECOD using NMISS();
proc sql;
create table dc as
select unique 'ADAE' as domain,
  compbl("SUBJECTID / AEDECOD") as key_grp_vr length=50
 , case when nmiss(aedecod) >= 1 then 'FAIL: Required Variable
    has at least one Missing Values'
  else 'PASS: Required Variable Does Not have any Missing
     Values' end as dc_rslt label="Data Check Results For:" length=75
   from adae;
quit;

* ADAE.AEDECOD using $CTNMISS format;
* Character vars use $ctnmiss. format and the convert to
     numeric since cmiss() does not work;
* Non-missing to 1 and blank missing to dot missing;
proc format;
```

(*Continued*)

Example 3.2.1 (*Continued*): Missing Values in Required Variable

```
value $ctnmiss ' ' = '.'
            other = '1';
value $ctmiss ' ' = 'Missing';
value nmiss . = 'Missing'
     other = 'Non-Missing';
QUIT;


proc sql;
create table dc as
select unique 'ADAE' as domain,
  compbl("SUBJECTID / AEDECOD") as key_grp_vr length=50
, case when nmiss(input(put(AEDECOD, $ctnmiss.), best.))
    >= 1 then 'FAIL: Required Variable has Missing Values'
  else 'PASS: Required Variable Does Not have Missing
    Values' end as dc_rslt label="Data Check Results For:" length=75
  from adae;
quit;
```

The results below show PASS for ADAE.ASTDT but FAILED for ADAE. AENDT. ADSL.AGE passed along with ADAE.AEDECOD using both methods. Once these high-level issues are found, detail records can then be sent to data management for query.

Output

Obs	domain	key_grp_vr	dc_rslt
1	ADAE	SUBJECTID / ASTDT	PASS: Required Variable Does Not have any Missing Values

Page Break

Obs	domain	key_grp_vr	dc_rslt
1	ADAE	SUBJECTID / AENDT	FAIL: Required Variable has at least one Missing Values

Page Break

Obs	domain	key_grp_vr	dc_rslt
1	ADSL	SUBJECTID / AGE	PASS: Required Variable Does Not have any Missing Values

Page Break

Obs	domain	key_grp_vr	dc_rslt
1	ADAE	SUBJECTID / AEDECOD	PASS: Required Variable Does Not have any Missing Values

Page Break

Obs	domain	key_grp_vr	dc_rslt
1	ADAE	SUBJECTID / AEDECOD	PASS: Required Variable Does Not have Missing Values

The next two examples check for missing values for permissible variables. The second example creates a test variable with all missing values.

Example 3.2.2: Missing Values in Permissible Variable

```
* Permissible variable with all missing values check;
* One record if any non-missing values and one record if any
    missing values;
proc sql;
create table dc as
select unique 'ADAE' as domain,
  compbl("SUBJECTID / aestdy") as key_grp_vr length=50
  , case when put(aestdy, nmiss.) = 'Missing' then 'Permissible
    Variable has Missing Values'
      when put(aestdy, nmiss.) = 'Non-Missing' then 'Permissible
        Variable has Non-Missing Values' end as dc_rslt
        label="Data Check Results For:" length=200
  from adae;
quit;

 * Condition test to show all missing values;
data ae1;
set ae;
permissible = .;
run;

proc sql;
create table dc as
select unique 'ADAE' as domain,
  compbl("SUBJECTID / permissible") as key_grp_vr length=50
  , case when put(permissible, nmiss.) = 'Missing' then 'Pemissible
    Variable has Missing Values'
      when put(permissible, nmiss.) = 'Non-Missing' then 'Permissble
        Variable has Non-Missing Values' end as dc_rslt label="Data
        Check Results For:" length=200
  from ae1;
quit;
```

Proc SQL's unique option displays only one record for each CASE instead of for each record. The first result shows AESTDY permissible variable has missing and non-missing values. The second result shows ADAE test variable PERMISSBLE variable has all missing values.

Output

Page Break

Obs	domain	key_grp_vr	dc_rslt
1	ADAE	SUBJECTID / aestdy	Permissible Variable has Missing Values
2	ADAE	SUBJECTID / aestdy	Permissible Variable has Non-Missing Values

Page Break

Obs	domain	key_grp_vr	dc_rslt
1	ADAE	SUBJECTID / permissible	Pemissible Variable has Missing Values

3.3 VARIABLE UNIQUE COUNTS

The variable unique count check frequency counts each unique value similar to using Proc FREQ. This confirms all unique values from the case report form exist in SDTMs. Proc FORMAT applies a missing label instead of a blank value in results. The second Proc SQL code creates counts for all records, non-missing records, unique row records and any missing records. Since the last two counts are the same, there are no missing SEX values. These are all useful dataset vitals.

Example 3.3.1: Variable Unique Counts

```
proc format;
value $ctmiss ' ' = 'Missing';
run;
proc sql;
create table dc as
select 'ADSL' as domain, put(sex, $ctmiss.) as sex1, count(*) as cnt
 from adsl group by calculated sex1;
quit;

* Alternative to Unit variable counts;
* Include all rows, with COUNT(*) notice that this isn't really
    specific to column A.;
* Include only non-missing values, with COUNT(A).;
```

(*Continued*)

Example 3.3.1 (*Continued*): Variable Unique Counts

```
* Exclude not only missing values, but also duplicate values, with
    COUNT(DISTINCT A).;
* Exclude duplicates, but include missing values (except, of
    course, duplicate missing values).;
proc sql;
create table dc as
select 'ADSL' as domain, 'SEX' as keyvar
    , count(*) as all_rows, count(sex) as non_missing_rows
    , count(distinct sex) as unique_rows
    , count(distinct sex) + max(missing(sex)) as unique_rows_
        plus_missing
  from adsl;
quit;
```

The first result shows 64 females and 123 males as two rows since it is GROUP BY SEX. The second result shows 187 total records, 0 missing and 2 unique SEX values as one row.

Output

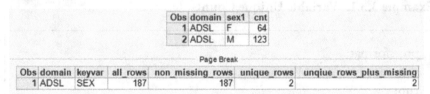

Obs	domain	sex1	cnt
1	ADSL	F	64
2	ADSL	M	123

Page Break

Obs	domain	keyvar	all_rows	non_missing_rows	unique_rows	unqiue_rows_plus_missing
1	ADSL	SEX	187	187	2	2

3.4 ISO8601 DATETIME AND TIME

ISO8601 datetime and time checks confirm all SDTM character date time format variables follow ISO8601 rules. The benefit of SDTMs having character date variables is to allow for raw partial date and time values. In the example below, there are two datasets, DCA and DCB. In DCA, the BAD_VALUE is created based on conditions to identify incorrect datetime values and is set to 1 for any record with bad values. The advantage of this approach is that DCA identifies which records fail the check based on BAD_VALUE being 1, and DCB identifies the overall check. Only the key variables are saved in DCA to focus on the check values. The condition to set failed records to 1 is within the CASE block with LENGTH() and INPUT() functions. Passed records are set to missing for BAD_VALUE. DCB uses summary functions on DCA to count the number of records with BAD_VALUE = 1. Note that SAS has specific ISO8601 formats that can be applied in these checks.

Example 3.4.1: ISO8601 Datetime and Time

```
data lb1;
set lb;
* test case;
*if _n_ = 1 then lbdtc = '2017-13-01';
run;

proc sql;
  create table dca as
  select a.usubjid, a.lbdtc,
  case when length(lbdtc) = 10 and input(lbdtc, is8601da.) = . then 1
  else . end as bad_value label='NOT Valid Date'
  from lb1 as a;

create table dcb as
select unique 'LB' as domain,
  compbl("SUBJECTID / lbdtc") as key_grp_vr length=50
  , case when count(bad_value) = 0 then 'PASS: Date format is
    valid'
  else 'FAIL: Date format is Not valid' end as dc_rslt label="Data
    Check Results For:" length=75
  from dca;
quit;

* Condition check for valid date, xxxdt ^= INPUT(xxDTC,
  E8601DA.);
* assure if only date then no T00:00;
data lb1;
set lb;
if _n_ = 1 then lbdtc = '2017-13-01T00:00:00';
run;
proc sql;
```

(*Continued*)

Example 3.4.1 (*Continued*): ISO8601 Datetime and Time

```
    create table dca as
    select a.usubjid, a.lbdtc,
    case when length(lbdtc) = 16 and find(lbdtc, 'T00:00') then 1
    else . end as bad_value label='FAIL: NOT Valid Date format'
    from lb1 as a;

create table dcb as
select unique 'LB' as domain,
 compbl("SUBJECTID / lbdtc") as key_grp_vr length=50
, case when count(bad_value) = 0 then 'PASS: Date is valid format'
else 'FAIL: Date format is Not valid' end as dc_rslt label="Data
  Check Results For:" length=75
 from dca;
quit;

* Condition check for valid datetime, treat dtc as valid dt - error
   if not valid datetime;
* e8601dt19. for extended formats '-' instead of base formats or
   is8601dt?;
data lb1;
set lb;
if _n_ = 1 then lbdtc = '2017-12-01T11:10';
if _n_ = 2 then lbdtc = '2017-12-01T99:10';
run;

proc sql;
 create table dca as
  select a.usubjid, a.lbdtc,
  case when length(lbdtc) = 16 and input(lbdtc, e8601dt19.) = . then 1
  else . end as bad_value label='FAIL: NOT Valid Date Time format'
  from lb1 as a;

create table dcb as
select unique 'LB' as domain,
 compbl("SUBJECTID / lbdtc") as key_grp_vr length=50
, case when count(bad_value) = 0 then 'PASS: Date Time format
  is valid'
```

(*Continued*)

Example 3.4.1 (*Continued*): ISO8601 Datetime and Time

```
  else 'FAIL: Date Time format is Not valid' end as dc_rslt
    label="Data Check Results For:" length=75
   from dca;
  quit;

  * Condition check for valid time, treat dtc as valid tm - error if
    not valid time;
  *    xxxtm ^= TIMEPART(xxxdtm);
  data lb1;
  set lb;
  if _n_ = 1 then lbdtc = '2017-12-01T11:10';
  if _n_ = 2 then lbdtc = '2017-12-01T99:10';
  run;

  proc sql;
   create table dca as
    select a.usubjid, a.lbdtc,
    case when length(lbdtc) = 16 and input(lbdtc, is8601dt.) = . then 1
    when length(lbdtc) = 8 and input(lbdtc, is8601tm.) = . then 1
    else . end as bad_value label='FAIL: NOT Valid Time format'
    from lb1 as a;

   create table dcb as
   select unique 'LB' as domain,
    compbl("SUBJECTID / lbdtc") as key_grp_vr length=50
   , case when count(bad_value) = 0 then 'PASS: Time format is
     valid'
   else 'FAIL: Time format is Not valid' end as dc_rslt label="Data
     Check Results For:" length=75
    from dca;
  quit;
```

The first DCB example PASSes ISO8601 requirements, but the next three DCB test results FAILed the ISO8601 requirements. This means that either the date or time was invalid of the ISO8601 format was not applied. DCA datasets store USUBJID, LBDTC and BAD_VALUE only so that it is easier to view data issues.

Output

Obs	domain	key_grp_vr	dc_rslt
1	LB	SUBJECTID / lbdtc	PASS: Date format is valid

Page Break

Obs	domain	key_grp_vr	dc_rslt
1	LB	SUBJECTID / lbdtc	FAIL: Date format is Not valid

Page Break

Obs	domain	key_grp_vr	dc_rslt
1	LB	SUBJECTID / lbdtc	FAIL: Date Time format is Not valid

Page Break

Obs	domain	key_grp_vr	dc_rslt
1	LB	SUBJECTID / lbdtc	FAIL: Time format is Not valid

3.5 DURATION

The duration check confirms consistency between duration variable and start and end date or time variables. This is ideal when the duration variable is collected on the case report form or when duration is calculated in ADaMs. DCA identifies which records fail, and DCB identifies the overall check. The second example is useful to expand each record with a starting and ending study day to one record per study day. The BAD_VALUE variable is defined as valid both start and end datetimes but calculated duration not equal to duration variable.

Example 3.5.1: Duration

```
data ae1;
set ae;
if _n_ = 1 then do; aestdtm = '2017-12-01T09:00'; aeendtm = '2017-
    12-01T09:25'; aedur=30;end;
CALL IS8601_CONVERT('dt/dt', 'du', aestdtm, aeendtm, aedur1);
run;

proc sql;
  create table dca as
```

(Continued)

Example 3.5.1 (*Continued*): Duration

```
    select a.usubjid, a.aestdtm, a.aeendtm, a.aedur,
    case when length(aestdtm) = 16 and length(aeendtm) = 16  and
    aedur1^= aedur then 1
    else . end as bad_value label='FAIL: NOT Valid Duration'
    from ae1 as a;

create table dcb as
select unique 'AE' as domain,
  compbl("SUBJECTID / aestdtm, aeendtm, aedur") as key_grp_
    vr length=50
, case when count(bad_value) = 0 then 'PASS: Duration is valid'
  else 'FAIL: Duration is Not valid' end as dc_rslt label="Data
    Check Results For:" length=75
  from dca;
quit;


* Expand from one record ae start and stop date to multiple
    records which will be one record per visit date;
* Assure only non-missing study days;
proc sort data=adae out=adae1;
by usubjid;
where nmiss(aestdy, aeendy) = 0;
run;

data dc;
set adae1;
 by usubjid;
keep usubjid aestdy aeendy ady ;
do i=aestdy to aeendy;
  ady=i;
output;
end;
run;
```

In AE, duration is FAILed, meaning it is not consistent with AE start and end date times. The second result DC dataset displays one record for each new study day value.

Output

Obs	domain	key_grp_vr	dc_rslt
1	AE	SUBJECTID / aestdtm, aeendtm, aedur	FAIL: Duration is Not valid

Obs	USUBJID	AESTDY	AEENDY	ady
1	███████	-21	-11	-21
2	███████	-21	-11	-20
3	███████	-21	-11	-19
4	███████	-21	-11	-18
5	███████	-21	-11	-17

3.6 DATA RANGE

Data range checks valid values by confirming all values are within the minimum and maximum acceptable values. There are many variables where this check can be applied for data quality. DCA identifies which records fail, and DCB identifies the overall check. The PASS message indicates that AGE values are within 0 and 100. The BAD_VALUE variable is based on ^ (Valid condition).

Example 3.6.1: Data Range

```
proc sql;
create table dca as
  select a.usubjid, a.age,
  case when ^(age is null or 0 <= age <= 100) then 1
  else . end as bad_value label='FAIL: NOT 0 <= AGE <= 100'
  from adsl as a;

create table dcb as
select unique 'ADSL' as domain,
  compbl("SUBJECTID / 0 <= AGE <= 100") as key_grp_vr length=50
  , case when count(bad_value) = 0 then 'PASS: Values Do Not Exist
    Outside of Range'
  else 'FAIL: Values Exist Outside of Range' end as dc_rslt label="Data
    Check Results For:" length=75
  from dca;
quit;
```

DCB displays valid AGE values between 0 and 100.

Output

Obs	domain	key_grp_vr	dc_rslt
1	ADSL	SUBJECTID / 0 <= AGE <= 100	PASS: Values Do Not Exist Outside of Range

3.7 NEGATIVE VALUES

The negative value check confirms non-negative values in selected variables. DCA identifies which records fail, and DCB identifies the overall check. The PASS message indicates all AGE values are greater than 0.

Example 3.7.1: Negative Value

```
proc sql;
create table dca as
  select a.usubjid, a.age,
  case when ^(0 < age) and age > . then 1
  else . end as bad_value label='FAIL: NOT AGE > 0'
  from adsl as a;

create table dcb as
select unique 'ADSL' as domain,
  compbl("SUBJECTID / 0 < AGE") as key_grp_vr length=50
  , case when count(bad_value) = 0 then 'PASS: Values Are
    Not Negative'
  else 'FAIL: Values Are Negative ' end as dc_rslt label="Data
    Check Results For:" length=75
  from dca;
quit;
```

DBC displays that AGE does not have any negative values.

Output

Obs	domain	key_grp_vr	dc_rslt
1	ADSL	SUBJECTID / 0 < AGE	PASS: Values Are Not Negative

3.8 NUMERIC OUTLIERS

Numeric outlier checks confirm that data assumptions are valid. Numeric outliers can skew the data, which impacts final statistical conclusions. In general, there are several methods to identify numeric outliers. Proc UNIVARIATE's NEXTROBS=10 option, for example, displays the top 10 extreme values. Proc FREQ can be used to sort and order data to show extreme small and large values. Proc SQL can also be used to count unique values and then sort to identify outliers. Finally, Proc RANK has options to rank and identify potential outliers.

Example 3.8.1: Numeric Outliers

```
ods output extremeobs=top10values;
proc univariate data=lb nextrobs=10;
var lbstresn;
id usubjid;
by lbtestcd;
run;
ods output close;

* Repeat for ADSL;
ods output extremeobs=top10values;
proc univariate data=adsl nextrobs=10;
var age;
id usubjid;
run;
ods output close;

* Repeat for AE top 10% aeterms;
* Summarize by aeterm;
proc sql;
create table ae1 as
select aeterm, count(usubjid) as aeterm_cnt from ae where aeterm
    > " group by aeterm;
quit;
```

(Continued)

Example 3.8.1 (*Continued*): Numeric Outliers

```
ods output extremeobs=top10values;
proc univariate data=ae1 nextrobs=10;
var aeterm_cnt;
id aeterm;
run;
ods output close;

* Top ten percent values by rank;
proc rank data=lb groups=10 out=top10percent (where =(r_lbstresn
   >= 9));
var lbstresn;
by lbtestcd;
ranks r_lbstresn;
run;

* Repeat for ADSL;
proc rank data=adsl groups=10 out=top10percent (where =(r_age
   >= 9));
var age;
ranks r_age;
run;

* Repeat for AE top 10% aeterms;
* Summarize by aeterm;
proc sql;
create table ae1 as
select aeterm, count(usubjid) as aeterm_cnt from ae where aeterm
   > " group by aeterm;
quit;

proc rank data=ae1 groups=10 out=top10percent (where =(r_aeterm_
   cnt >= 9));
var aeterm_cnt;
ranks r_aeterm_cnt;
run;
```

(*Continued*)

Example 3.8.1 (*Continued*): Numeric Outliers

```
* Edit check to watch out for disproportionate number of lows or
    highs;
data lb1;
set lb;
if _n_ <= 25 then RNGFLAG = 'L';
else RNGFLAG = 'H';
run;


PROC SORT DATA = LB1 out=lb2;
BY lbtestcd;
RUN;


* Inbalance of normal flags - L and H;
* Count the number of Ls, Ns, and Hs;
* consider nlevels option to display nlevels, nmisslevels and
    nnonmisslevel vars;
PROC FREQ DATA = LB2 NOPRINT;
BY Lbtestcd;
WHERE RNGFLAG NE ' ';
TABLE RNGFLAG / OUT=dca;
RUN;


* Take a look at Ls and Hs that occur more than 75% of the time;
DATA dcb;
set dca;
IF RNGFLAG IN ('L','H') AND PERCENT GE 75 ;
RUN;
```

The sample results display extreme values from Proc UNIVARIATE.

Output

The UNIVARIATE Procedure
Variable: LBSTRESN (Numeric Result/Finding in Standard Units)

Lab Test or Examination Short Name=BCELL

Moments			
N	1	Sum Weights	1
Mean	0.05086628	Sum Observations	0.05086628
Std Deviation	.	Variance	.
Skewness	.	Kurtosis	.
Uncorrected SS	0.00258738	Corrected SS	0
Coeff Variation	.	Std Error Mean	.

Basic Statistical Measures			
Location		Variability	
Mean	0.050866	Std Deviation	.
Median	0.050866	Variance	.
Mode	0.050866	Range	0
		Interquartile Range	0

Tests for Location: Mu0=0			
Test	Statistic	p Value	
Student's t	t	.	Pr > |t|	.
Sign	M	0.5	Pr >= |M|	1.0000
Signed Rank	S	0.5	Pr >= |S|	1.0000

Quantiles (Definition 5)

3.9 COMPARE RELATED VARIABLES

The compare related variables check confirm logically, consistency and integrity across variables within and across SDTMs. After applying unit-level checks, comparing related variables checks is essential for high-quality submissions since inconsistent variables are often easier to detect. Inconsistencies can happen between start and end dates or any related variables. Many of the examples in this section are based on rules between two or more variables that must all be non-missing, missing or be logically and mathematically correct. The DCA and DCB dataset methods work well to identify any issues at the record level as well as at the summary level. DCA dataset contains only the variables checked to make it easier to identify data issues.

The example below confirms sequence of ADAE start and end date variables with the condition to first confirm both dates are non-missing and then a not condition on start date same or before end date. It is important to double check that both dates are non-missing when comparing dates; otherwise, check results may not make sense.

Example 3.9.1: Sequence of ADAE Start and End Date Variables

```
proc sql;
create table dca as
  select a.usubjid, a.ASTDT, a.AENDT,
  case when nmiss(ASTDT, AENDT)=0 and ^(ASTDT <=
  AENDT) then 1
  else . end as bad_value label='FAIL: NOT ASTDT <= AENDT'
  from adae as a;

create table dcb as
select unique 'ADAE' as domain,
  compbl("usubjid / ASTDT <= AENDT") as key_grp_vr length=50
  , case when count(bad_value) = 0 then 'PASS: Variables are
    Not Inconsistent'
  else 'FAIL: Variables are Inconsistent' end as dc_rslt label="Data
    Check Results For:" length=75
  from dca;
quit;
```

DCB shows PASS for all ADAE start dates are same of before the end dates. DCB contains USUBJID, ASTDT, AENDT and BAD_VALUE.

Output

Obs	domain	key_grp_vr	dc_rslt
1	ADAE	usubjid / ASTDT <= AENDT	PASS: Variables are Not Inconsistent

The example below confirms AE start date is the same or before the DS disposition date. CMISS() function is used to confirm both dates are non-missing. The Proc SQL code uses NMISS() to confirm non-missing dates and then^(valid condition) to indentify BAD_VABLUE flag.

Example 3.9.2: Sequence of AE Start Date and DS Date Variables

```
proc sql;
create table ae_ds as
  select a.*, b.*
  from ae as a, ds as b where a.usubjid = b.usubjid;

create table dca as
  select a.usubjid, a.AEsTDTc, a.dsstdtc,
  case when cmiss(AESTDTc, dsstdtc)=0 and ^(input(AeSTDTc,
    is8601da.) <= input(dsstdtc, is8601da.)) then 1
  else . end as bad_value label='NOT AeSTDTc <= dsstdtc'
  from ae_ds as a;

create table dcb as
select unique 'AE' as domain,
  compbl("usubjid / AESTDTc <= dsstdtc") as key_grp_vr
    length=50
  , case when count(bad_value) = 0 then 'PASS: Variables are
    Not Inconsistent'
  else 'FAIL: Variables are Inconsistent' end as dc_rslt label="Data
    Check Results For:" length=75
from dca;
quit;
```

DCB shows FAIL that at least one AE start date is not the same or before the DS disposition date. DCA can then be reviewed to identify which patient had this data issue.

Output

Obs	domain	key_grp_vr	dc_rslt
1	AE	usubjid / AeSTDTc <= dsstdtc	FAIL: Variables are Inconsistent

The example below confirms multivariate non-missing values for AEDECOD and AEPTCD.

Example 3.9.3: AE Multivariate Non-Missing for AEDECOD and AEPTCD

```
proc sql;
create table dca as
  select a.usubjid, a.aedecod, a.aeptcd,
  case when cmiss(aedecod, aeptcd) = 1 then 1
  else . end as bad_value label='FAIL: Not Both Missing or
    Non-Missing AEDECOD, AEPTCD'
  from ae as a;

create table dcb as
select unique 'AE' as domain,
  compbl("SUBJECTID / AEDECOD and AEPTCD") as key_grp_
    vr length=50
, case when count(bad_value) = 0 then 'PASS: Variables are Not
    Inconsistent (Missing/Non-missing)'
  else 'FAIL: Variables are Inconsistent (Missing/Non-missing)'
    end as dc_rslt label="Data Check Results For:" length=75
  from dca;
quit;
```

DCB shows PASS for both AEDECOD and AEPTCD consistently missing or non-missing.

Output

Obs	domain	key_grp_vr	dc_rslt
1	AE	SUBJECTID / AEDECOD and AEPTCD	PASS: Variables are Not Inconsistent (Missing/Non-missing)

The example below confirms multivariate non-missing check for CLASS dataset.

Example 3.9.4: Class Multivariate Non-Missing for WEIGHT and HEIGHT

```
proc sql;
create table dca as
   select  a.name, a.weight, a.height,
   case when nmiss(weight, height)=1 then 1
   else . end as bad_value label='FAIL: Not Both Missing or
      Non-Missing WEIGHT, HEIGHT'
   from sashelp.class as a;

create table dcb as
select unique 'CLASS' as domain,
   compbl("SUBJECTID / WEIGHT HEIGHT") as key_grp_vr
      length=50
, case when count(bad_value) = 0 then 'PASS: Variables are
      Not Inconsistent (Missing/Non-missing)'
   else 'FAIL: Variables are Inconsistent (Missing/Non-missing)'
      end as dc_rslt label="Data Check Results For:" length=75
   from dca;
quit;
```

DCB shows PASS for WEIGHT and HEIGHT consistently being both missing or non-missing.

Output

Obs	domain	key_grp_vr	dc_rslt
1	CLASS	SUBJECTID / WEIGHT HEIGHT	PASS: Variables are Not Inconsistent (Missing/Non-missing)

The example below confirms multivariate non-missing check for LB. Proc FORMAT creates the $CTNMISS format, which converts all missing values to '.' so it is displayed and all other non-missing values to '1'. This will be applied to LBSTRESC to collapse all values into two categories – missing and non-missing. This is important to confirm both LBSTRESC and LBSRESN are non-missing for the same record. The N() and INPUT() functions are applied with $CTNMISS format to set BAD_VALUE = 1 for failed records.

Example 3.9.5: LB Multivariate Non-Missing for LBSTRESC and LBSTRESN

```
* Inconsistent char and numeric lab vars, ie one missing -
    lbstresc lbstresn;
* convert char to numeric with format and put and input
    functions;
* or for mixed case use char = " and num = .;
proc format;
value $ctnmiss ' ' = '.'
    other = '1';
quit;

proc sql;
create table dca as
   select a.usubjid, a.lbstresc, a.lbstresn,
   case when n(lbstresn, input(put(lbstresc, $ctnmiss.), best.))
   = 1 then 1
   else . end as bad_value label='FAIL: Not Both Missing or
   Non-Missing lbstresc lbstresn'
   from lb as a;

create table dcb as
select unique 'LB' as domain,
   compbl("SUBJECTID / lbstresc lbstresn") as key_grp_vr
   length=50
   , case when count(bad_value) = 0 then 'PASS: Variables are
   Not Inconsistent (Missing/Non-missing)'
   else 'FAIL: Variables are Inconsistent (Missing/Non-missing)'
   end as dc_rslt label="Data Check Results For:" length=75
   from dca;
quit;
```

DCB shows FAIL for LBSTRESC and LBSTRESN consistently being both missing or non-missing. This check documents that at least one of the two variables is missing and the other is non-missing. DCA can be reviewed to identify the failed records by viewing USUBJID, LBSTRESC, LBSTRESN and BAD_VALUE.

Output

Obs	domain	key_grp_vr	dc_rslt
1	LB	SUBJECTID / lbstresc lbstresn	FAIL: Variables are Inconsistent (Missing/Non-missing)

As an alternative to the previous example, the example below also confirms multivariate non-missing value but for missing values of LBSTRESC and non-missing values of LBSTRESN. This is a one-sided test since it does not check for missing LBSTRESN and non-missing LBSTRESC.

Example 3.9.6: LB Multivariate Non-Missing for LBSTRESC and LBSTRESN

```
* Repeat for Missing unit (char) for non-missing lab value (num)
   - lbstresu lbstresn;

* Missing char result for non-missing lab value (num) - lbstresc
   lbstresn;
proc sql;
create table dca as
   select a.usubjid, a.lbstresc, a.lbstresn,
   case when lbstresn > . and lbstresc = '' then 1
   else . end as bad_value label='FAIL: Missing CHAR LBSTRESC
   and Non-Missing NUM LBSTRESN'
   from lb as a;

create table dcb as
select unique 'LB' as domain,
   compbl("SUBJECTID / lbstresc lbstresn") as key_grp_vr
   length=50
   , case when count(bad_value) = 0 then 'PASS: Not Missing
   CHAR LBSTRESC and Non-Missing NUM LBSTRESN'
   else 'FAIL: Missing CHAR LBSTRESC and Non-Missing
   NUM LBSTRESN)' end as dc_rslt label="Data Check Results
   For:" length=75
   from dca;
quit;
```

DCB shows PASS for LBSTRESC and LBSTRESN consistently being both missing or non-missing.

Output

Obs	domain	key_grp_vr	dc_rslt
1	LB	SUBJECTID / lbstresc lbstresn	PASS: Not Missing CHAR LBSTRESC and Non-Missing NUM LBSTRESN

The example below confirms multivariate value for AE. AEENDTC should be missing for AEENRTPT = ONGOING.

Example 3.9.7: AE Multivariate for AEENRTPT = 'ONGOING' and AEENDTC

```
proc sql;
create table dca as
   select a.usubjid, a.aeenrtpt, a.AEENDTC,
   case when AEENDTC ='' and ^(aeenrtpt='ONGOING') then 1
   else . end as bad_value label='FAIL: NOT aeenrtpt=ONGOING
      and AEENDTC blank'
   from ae as a;


create table dcb as
select unique 'AE' as domain,
 compbl("SUBJECTID / aeenrtpt=ONGOING and AEENDTC
    blank") as key_grp_vr length=75
, case when count(bad_value) = 0 then'PASS: Variables are
   Not Inconsistent'
else 'FAIL: Variables are Inconsistent' end as dc_rslt label="Data
   Check Results For:" length=50
 from dca;
quit;
```

A similar check can be applied for the following multivariate conditions:

- LBSTAT = 'NOT DONE' and LBORRES non-missing.
- LBSTAT ^= 'NOT DONE' and LBORRES missing.
- AESTDY/AEENDY non-missing for each AESTDTC/AEENDTC.
- AESTDT/CMSTDT missing and AEENDT/CMENDT non-missing.
- AESDTH^='Y' and AEOUT='FATAL'.
- If CMOCCUR='N' and CMENRF and CMENDTC non-missing.
- Screen failure and ARM non-missing.
- AE Terms before dose day 1 are study drug^='NOT RELATED'.
- AE Event leads to death and death date missing.
- AE Event leads to dose interruption or reduction and dose is not consistent.
- End of treatment disposition not consistent with tumor assessment, ex. both disease progression.
- Number of assessments on target, non-target and response are not consistent.
- AEYN = 'Yes' and AESPID missing.
- RESULTC non-missing and length(RESULTC) ne 11.
- DCCHANGE = 'No' and DCINDOSE ne DCADDOSE.
- EGNA missing and EGYN ne 'No'.
- ADCM.ASTDTF non-missing and ASTDT missing.
- NOT (EX.EXSTDY > EXENDY > .z).
- NOT((SAFFL= 'Y' and SAFFN=1) or (SAFFL= 'N' and SAFFN=0) or (SAFFL= "and SAFFN=.)).
- AEOUT is not 'FATAL' and AESDTH= 'Y'.
- VISIT inconsistent with VISITNUM.

The DCB results show PASS for both AEENTRPT='ONGOING' and AEENDTC missing.

Output

Obs	domain	key_grp_vr	dc_rslt
1	AE	SUBJECTID / aeenrtpt=ONGOING and AEENDTC blank	PASS: Variables are Not Inconsistent

The example below confirms multivariate checks for CLASS comparing two numeric variables.

Example 3.9.8: Class Multivariate for WEIGHT and HEIGHT

```
* Condition test since weight will most likely be > height;
proc sql;
create table dca as
  select a.name, a.weight, a.height,
  case when nmiss(weight, height)=0 and ^(weight < height) then 1
  else . end as bad_value label='FAIL: NOT WEIGHT < HEIGHT'
  from sashelp.class as a;

create table dcb as
select unique 'CLASS' as domain,
 compbl("SUBJECTID / WEIGHT < HEIGHT") as key_grp_vr
   length=50
, case when count(bad_value) = 0 then 'PASS: Variables are
  Not Inconsistent'
else 'FAIL: Variables are Inconsistent' end as dc_rslt label="Data
  Check Results For:" length=75
 from dca;
quit;
```

DCB shows FAIL for WEIGHT < HEIGHT. The DCA dataset can then be reviewed to identify which name had this data issue.

Output

Obs	domain	key_grp_vr	dc_rslt
1	CLASS	SUBJECTID / WEIGHT < HEIGHT	FAIL: Variables are Inconsistent

The example below confirms multivariate values for AESER to be 'Y' if at least one of these exist, AESDTH, AESLIFE or AESHOSP.

Example 3.9.9: AE Multivariate for AESER

```
proc sql;
create table dca as
  select a.usubjid, a.AESLIFE, a.AESHOSP, a.AESER,
  case when AESER='Y' and ^(AESLIFE='Y' or AESHOSP='Y')
  then 1
  else . end as bad_value label='FAIL: NOT AESDTH AESLIFE
  AESHOSP AESER'
  from ae as a;

create table dcb as
select unique 'AE' as domain,
  compbl("SUBJECTID / AESLIFE, AESHOSP, AESER") as key_
  grp_vr length=50
  , case when count(bad_value) = 0 then 'PASS: Variables are
  Not Inconsistent'
  else 'FAIL: Variables are Inconsistent' end as dc_rslt label="Data
  Check Results For:" length=75
  from dca;
quit;
```

DCB shows PASS for AESLIFE, AESHOSP and AESER are consistent.
DCB stores USUBJID, AESLIFE, AESHOSP, AESER and BAD_VALUE.

Output

Obs	domain	key_grp_vr	dc_rslt
1	AE	SUBJECTID / AESLIFE, AESHOSP, AESER	PASS: Variables are Not Inconsistent

The example below confirms multivariate values for AETOXGR = 5 for AESLIFE='Y'.

Example 3.9.10: AE Multivariate for AETOXGR and AELIFE

```
proc sql;
create table dca as
  select a.usubjid, a.AETOXGR, a.AESLIFE,
  case when AETOXGR='5' and ^(AESLIFE='Y') then 1
  else . end as bad_value label='FAIL: NOT AETOXGR and
    AESLIF'
  from ae as a;

create table dcb as
select unique 'AE' as domain,
  compbl("SUBJECTID / AETOXGR, AESLIFE") as key_grp_vr
  length=50
  , case when count(bad_value) = 0 then 'PASS: Variables are
  Not Inconsistent'
  else 'FAIL: Variables are Inconsistent' end as dc_rslt label="Data
    Check Results For:" length=75
  from dca;
quit;
```

DCB shows PASS for AETOXGR and AELIFE are consistent.

Output

Obs	domain	key_grp_vr	dc_rslt
1	AE	SUBJECTID / AETOXGR, AESLIFE	PASS: Variables are Not Inconsistent

The example below confirms multivariate values AESLIFE = 'Y' and DM.DTHFL='Y'. The first Proc SQL LEFT JOINs AE with DM to keep all AE records. The second Proc SQL takes the max values of AESLIFE and DTHFL GROUP BY USUBJID to identify non-missing values.

Example 3.9.11: AE Multivariate for AE.AESLIFE and DM.DTHFL

```
proc sql;
create table dca as
    select unique a.usubjid, a.AESLIFE, b.DTHFL,
    case when a.AESLIFE='Y' and ^(b.DTHFL = 'Y') then 1
    when a.AESLIFE ^='Y' and (b.DTHFL = 'Y') then 1
    else . end as bad_value label='FAIL: NOT AE.AESLIFE and
        DM.DTHFL'
    from ae as a left join dm as b on a.usubjid=b.usubjid;

create table dcb as
    select unique a.usubjid, max(a.AESLIFE) as aeslife, max(a.
        DTHFL) as dthfl,
    max(bad_value) as bad_value
    from dca as a group by usubjid;

create table dcc as
select unique 'AE' as domain,
    compbl("SUBJECTID / AE.AESLIFE, DM.DTHFL") as key_
        grp_vr length=50
    , case when count(bad_value) = 0 then 'PASS: Variables are
        Not Inconsistent'
    else 'FAIL: Variables are Inconsistent' end as dc_rslt
        label="Data Check Results For:" length=75
    from dcb;
quit;
```

The results show FAIL for AE.AESLIFE and DM.DTHFL are consistent.

Output

Obs	domain	key_grp_vr	dc_rslt
1	AE	SUBJECTID / AE.AESLIFE, DM.DTHFL	FAIL: Variables are Inconsistent

The example multivariate check below validates values for DM. RFSTDTC and RFENDTC should be non-missing if patient was randomized.

Example 3.9.12: DM Multivariate for RFSTDTC and ARMCD

```
proc sql;
create table dca as
   select a.usubjid, a.RFSTDTC, a.ARMCD,
   case when nmiss(ARMCD)=0 and ^(RFSTDTC > '') then 1
   else . end as bad_value label='FAIL: NOT RFSTDTC and
     ARMCD non-missing'
   from dm as a;

create table dcb as
select unique 'DM' as domain,
   compbl("usubjid / RFSTDTC, ARMCD") as key_grp_vr
   length=50
   , case when count(bad_value) = 0 then 'PASS: Variables are
   Not Inconsistent'
   else 'FAIL: Variables are Inconsistent' end as dc_rslt label="Data
   Check Results For:" length=75
   from dca;
quit;
```

The results show FAIL for RFSTDTC and ARMCD are consistent.

Output

Obs	domain	key_grp_vr	dc_rslt
1	DM	usubjid / RFSTDTC, ARMCD	FAIL: Variables are Inconsistent

3.10 CALCULATIONS AND DERIVED VARIABLE

This section shows calculations and derived variable checks. This consists of applying non-missing checks to both SDTM and derived variable. Also, if there is a difference between the derived and SDTM variable, then BAD_VALUE is set to 1.

The example below confirms DM AGE calculation by comparing it with AGE. Since age is dynamically created, the CALCULATED keyword must be placed before CK_AGE. This direct process works well for simple calculations such as AGE. For more complex calculations, the variable can be created and then compared using Proc SQL.

Example 3.10.1: Numeric Calculations

```
proc sql;
create table dca as
  select a.usubjid, a.tr01sdt, a.birthdt, a.age, floor((tr01sdt
    - birthdt)/365) as ck_age,
  case when nmiss(tr01sdt, birthdt) = 0 and abs(age - calculated
    ck_age) ^in (0, 1) then 1
  else . end as bad_value label='FAIL: Not FLOOR((tr01sdt
    - birthdt)/365)'
  from adsl as a;

create table dcb as
select unique 'ADSL' as domain,
  compbl("SUBJECTID / FLOOR(tr01sdt - birthdt)/365") as key_
    grp_vr length=50
, case when count(bad_value) = 0 then 'PASS: AGE Calculation
    Is Correct'
  else 'FAIL: AGE Calculation Is Not Correct' end as dc_rslt
    label="Data Check Results For:" length=75
  from dca;
quit;
```

The results show PASS for AGE calculation.

Output

Obs	domain	key_grp_vr	dc_rslt
1	ADSL	SUBJECTID / FLOOR(tr01sdt - birthdt)/365	PASS: AGE Calculation Is Correct

The example below confirms ADAE study day calculation. Since study day is derived within Proc SQL, CALCULATED is applied before CK_AESTDY to use CK_AESTDY in the CASE condition.

Example 3.10.2: Study Day

```
proc sql;
create table dca as
  select a.usubjid, a.astdt, a.tr01sdt, a.aestdy, (ASTDT - TR01SDT
    + (AStDT > TR01SDT)) as ck_aestdy,
  case when nmiss(astdt, tr01sdt) = 0 and abs(aestdy - calculated
    ck_aestdy) ^in (0, 1) then 1
  else . end as bad_value label='FAIL: Not ASTDT - TRTSDT +
    (AStDT > TRTSDT)'
  from adae as a;


create table dcb as
select unique 'ADAE' as domain,
  compbl("SUBJECTID / ASTDT – TRTSDT + (AStDT >
  TRTSDT)") as key_grp_vr length=50
  , case when count(bad_value) = 0 then 'PASS: Study Day Is
  Correct'
  else 'FAIL: Study Day Is Not Correct' end as dc_rslt label="Data
  Check Results For:" length=75
  from dca;
quit;
```

The results show PASS for ADAE start study day calculation.

Output

Obs	domain	key_grp_vr	dc_rslt
1	ADAE	SUBJECTID / ASTDT – TRTSDT + (AStDT > TRTSDT)	PASS: Study Day Is Correct

The example below confirms ADAE study day does not equal 0. This check can be applied to any domain with study day.

Example 3.10.3: Study Day

```
* Study day equal 0 check;
proc sql;
create table dca as
   select unique a.usubjid, a.aestdy, a.aeendy,
   case when aestdy =0 or aeendy=0 then 1
   else . end as bad_value label='FAIL: aestdy or aeendy = 0'
   from adae as a;

 create table dcb as
select unique 'ADAE' as domain,
  compbl("SUBJECTID / aestdy or  aeendy = 0)") as key_grp_vr
    length=50
  , case when count(bad_value) = 0 then 'PASS: Study Day Is
    Not Equal to Zero'
  else 'FAIL: Study Day Equals Zero' end as dc_rslt label="Data
    Check Results For:" length=75
   from dca;
quit;
```

The results show FAIL meaning that ADAE start or end study day equals an invalid 0.

Output

Obs	domain	key_grp_vr	dc_rslt
1	ADAE	SUBJECTID / aestdy or aeendy = 0)	FAIL: Study Day Equals Zero

3.11 LAB DATA

Lab data checks are critical since lab data can be over 70% of the raw data. The lab checks in this section focus on lab unit conversions, lab differentials and normal range checks.

The example below confirms lab unit conversions. For each LBTESTCD, there should be unique LBSTRESU values. Duplicate record count for LBTESTCD for LBSTRESU values indicate multiple units for the same LBTESTCD. This check can be repeated for paired variables such as TRTAGYN and TRTAGY.

DCA dataset stores USUBJID, LBDTC, LBTESTCD, LBSTRESU, LBSTRESN and DUPCNT grouped by LBTESTCD. DUPCNT is count of unique LBSTRESU values so ideally there is only a one-to-one correspondence between LBSTRESU and LBTESTCD. DCB counts the number of records by USUBJID to identify if check failed.

Example 3.11.1: Lab Unit Conversions

```
data lb1;
set lb;
if _n_ = 1 then do; lbstresu='#'; lbstresn=10; end;
run;

 proc sql;
  create table dca as
  select a.usubjid, a.lbdtc, a.lbtestcd, a.lbstresu, a.lbstresn, b.dupcnt
  from lb1 as a,
  (select count(unique lbstresu) as dupcnt label='Duplicate record
    count' from lb1 where lbstresn > . group by lbtestcd) as b;

  create table dcb as
  select unique 'LB' as domain,
    compbl("USUBJID / lbtestcd, lbstresu") as key_grp_vr
      length=50
    , case when count(usubjid) > 1 then 'FAIL: Duplicate Records Exist'
    else 'PASS: Duplicate Records Do Not Exist' end as dc_rslt
      label="Data Check Results For:" length=75
  from dca where dupcnt > 1;
  quit;
```

The results show FAIL because multiple values of LBSTRESU exist for the same LBTESTCD.

Output

Obs	domain	key_grp_vr	dc_rslt
1	LB	USUBJID / lbtestcd, lbstresu	FAIL: Duplicate Records Exist

The example below confirms special characters do not exist in lab data by comparing the character variable LBSTRESC with the numeric variable

LBSTRESN. With a combination of ANYALPHA() and ANYALNUM() functions, this example confirms only valid alpha character or numeric values exist. The first WHEN condition checks for numeric values and the second WHEN condition checks for alpha values. Check results are based on ^(valid condition).

Example 3.11.2: Special Characters in Lab Data

```
proc sql;
create table dca as
  select a.USUBJID, a.lbstresc, a.lbstresn,
  case when ^(anyalpha(trim(lbstresc)) = 0 and lbstresn=input
  (lbstresc, best8.)) then 1
    when ^(anyalnum(trim(lbstresc)) = 0 and lbstresn=.) then 1
    when lbstresc = " and lbstresn=. then 1
    else . end as bad_value label='FAIL: NOT lbstresc, lbstresn'
  from lb as a;

create table dcb as
select unique 'LB' as domain,
  compbl("USUBJID / lbstresc lbstresn") as key_grp_vr length=50
, case when count(bad_value) > 0 then 'PASS: Variables are
    Not Inconsistent'
else 'FAIL: Variables are Inconsistent' end as dc_rslt label="Data
    Check Results For:" length=75
from dca where lbstresc > " and bad_value > .;
quit;
```

The results show PASS for LBSTRESC and LBSTRESN are consistent.

Output

Obs	domain	key_grp_vr	dc_rslt
1	LB	USUBJID / lbstresc lbstresn	PASS: Variables are Not Inconsistent

The example below confirms values are left justified so that leading spaces do not exist. AETERM is compared with LEFT(AETERM) to set failed records with BAD_VALUE = 1.

Example 3.11.3: Character Variables Left Alignment

```
proc sql;
create table dca as
  select a.usubjid, a.aeterm,
  case when ^(aeterm = left(aeterm)) then 1
  else . end as bad_value label='FAIL: NOT Left AETERM'
  from adae as a;

create table dcb as
select unique 'ADAE' as domain,
  compbl("USUBJID / AETERM") as key_grp_vr length=50
  , case when count(bad_value) = 0 then 'PASS: Variable does
    Not have leading Blanks'
  else 'FAIL: Variable has leading blanks' end as dc_rslt
    label="Data Check Results For:" length=75
from dca;
quit;
```

The results show PASS for AETERM not having leading blanks.

Output

Obs	domain	key_grp_vr	dc_rslt
1	ADAE	USUBJID / AETERM	PASS: Variable does Not have leading Blanks

SUMMARY

This chapter provides a variety of data checks across several types of SDTMs and ADaMs. Essential checks including duplicate records, missing required variables and ISO8601 datetime and time checks can be applied across all SDTMs and, ADaMs. In addition, almost all SDTMs and ADaMs require a comparison between two or more related variables. While standardized control terms greatly help to review and analyze the data, data checks are still required since there are many opportunities for introducing programming or data error in the SDTM and ADaM creation process.

CHAPTER 4

CDISC Specification Compliance Checks

INTRODUCTION

CDISC specification compliance checks are applicable to both SDTMs and ADaMs. Examples of CDISC specification compliance checks include consistency among specifications and SDTM attributes and order of variables. The CDISC specification compliance checks must pass through Pinnacle 21 checks, which most organizations run at early stage to prevent late minute SDTM and ADaM updates before submission.

Below are examples of useful metadata checks:

- Length of any variable name > 8 characters

- Length of any variable label > 40 characters

- Length of any variable value > 200 characters

- Variable types other than character or numeric

- Presence of special characters in variable names

See Appendix Table A.8 for example of converting SDTM specifications into a dataset to be used as metadata. Many of the examples in this book use SDTM IG 3.2 version specifications.

4.1 CONSISTENCY BETWEEN DM SPECIFICATIONS AND ATTRIBUTES (TYPE, NAME, LENGTH, LABEL)

Consistency between DM specifications and attributes confirm the two files are in sync. The DM specification needs to be converted to a dataset so that metadata between the DM specifications and DM domain can be compared. See Proc IMPORT examples to convert Excel to datasets. The example below shows changing the SASHELP.CLASS dataset to directly compare datasets at three levels. The first Proc SQL compares metadata datasets.

Example 4.1.1: Consistency between Similar Domains

```
* Create sample datasets;
proc sort data=sashelp.class out=class;
by name;
run;

data class;
length Sex 8.;
set class (drop=sex);
sex=1;
age=10;
if _n_ <= 10;
keep name sex age;
run;

* 1 - physical metadata - compare of dataset file attributes;
proc sql;
  create table class_1 as
  select libname, memname, crdate, nobs, nvar, filesize
  from sashelp.vtable where upcase(libname) in ('SASHELP' 'WORK')
    and upcase(memname) in ('CLASS');
quit;

proc transpose data=class_1 out=class_2 (drop= _name_ _label_);
by memname;
id libname;
var crdate;
run;
```

The results show three levels: metadata datasets, metadata variable attributes and data values. As expected, the differences are displayed. The metadata dataset shows when the physical files were created and their size, as well as the number of observations and variables. This confirms data is transferred correctly between folders.

Output

Obs	libname	memname	crdate	nobs	nvar	filesize
1	WORK	CLASS	02FEB19:13:40:29	10	3	131072
2	SASHELP	CLASS	24JUN15:21:07:09	19	5	131072

The second example compares metadata variable attributes of CLASS from the SASHELP and WORK libraries. The first SQL creates a dataset similar to that of SDTM specifications of DM below. The Data Step merges the two CLASS datasets by NAME to flag any attribute differences. Once differences with DM specifications are identified, the DDT DM specification and domain can be updated to be in compliance.

VARIABLE	TYPE	LENGTH	LABEL
STUDYID	text	15	Study Identifier
DOMAIN	text	2	Domain Abbreviation
USUBJID	text	25	Unique Subject Identifier
SUBJID	text	7	Subject Identifier for the Study
RFSTDTC	date	16	Subject Reference Start Date/Time
RFENDTC	date	16	Subject Reference End Date/Time
SITEID	text	7	Study Site Identifier
BRTHDTC	date	16	Date/Time of Birth
AGE	integer	8	Age
AGEU	text	5	Age Units
SEX	text	2	Sex
RACE	text	40	Race
ARMCD	text	8	Planned Arm Code
ARM	text	40	Description of Planned Arm
COUNTRY	text	3	Country

Example 4.1.2: Consistency between Specifications and Dataset Attributes

```
* variable metadata - compare dataset attributes;
* This approach enables var by var comparison instead of record
   by record comparison if single proc sql;

proc sql;
 create table class_sashelp as
   select name, type, length, label, format
   from sashelp.vcolumn where upcase(libname) = 'SASHELP' and
      upcase(memname) = 'CLASS' order by name;
quit;

* domain dictionary table;
proc sql;
 create table class_work as
   select name, type as b_type, length as b_length, label as b_label,
      format as b_format
   from sashelp.vcolumn where libname = 'WORK' and
      upcase(memname) = 'CLASS' order by name;
quit;

data class_2;
merge class_sashelp (in=a) class_work (in=b);
by name;
if ^(a=b) or ^(type=b_type and length=b_length and label=b_
   label and format=b_format) then diff=1;
run;

proc sort data=class_2;
by descending diff;
run;
```

The results show differences in CLASS metadata variable attributes by DIFF=1.

<!-- Page Break -->

Obs	name	type	length	label	format	b_type	b_length	b_label	b_format	diff
1	Height	num	8				.			1
2	Sex	char	1			num	8			1
3	Weight	num	8				.			1
4	Age	num	8			num	8			.
5	Name	char	8			char	8			.

The third example applies Proc COMPARE to compare data values.

As an alternative to example 4.1.2, the example below also directly compares attributes from similar SDTMs. The LAG() function is helpful to compare TYPE, LENGTH, LABEL and FORMATs to identify any differences in FLAG.

```
proc sql;
   create table dc as
   select name, memname, type, length, label, format, count(name)
      as dupcnt
   from sashelp.vcolumn where upcase(libname) in ('SDTM') group
      by name having calculated dupcnt > 1;
quit;

proc sort datadata=dc;
by name memname;
run;

data dc1;
length lag_type $8. lag_length 8. lag_label $8. lag_format $8. flag $1.;
set dc;
by name memname;

lag_type=lag(type);  lag_length=lag(length);  lag_label=lag(label);
lag_format=lag(format);

if first.name then do;
   lag_type=type;  lag_length=length;  lag_label=label;  lag_
      format=format;
end;
   if last.name and lag_type^=: type or lag_length^=: length or
      lag_label^=: label or lag_format^=: format then flag='Y';
   drop lag_type lag_length lag_label lag_format;
run;

proc sort data= dc1 nodupkey out=lookup (keep= name);
by name;
where flag = 'Y';
run;
```

(*Continued*)

```
proc sql;
create table dc2 as
   select a.* from dc1 as a, lookup as b where a.name = b.name;
quit;

title 'Differneces in common vars';
proc print;run;
```

Differneces in common vars

Obs	flag	name	memname	type	length	label	format	dupcnt
1		Age	CLASSA	num	8			2
2		Age	CLASSB	num	8			2
3		Height	CLASSA	num	8			2
4		Height	CLASSB	num	8			2
5		Name	CLASSA	char	8			2
6		Name	CLASSB	char	8			2
7		Sex	CLASSA	char	1			2
8	Y	Sex	CLASSB	num	8			2
9		Weight	CLASSA	num	8			2
10		Weight	CLASSB	num	8			2
11		format	DC	char	49	Column Format		2
12		format	DC1	char	49	Column Format		2
13		label	DC	char	256	Column Label		2
14		label	DC1	char	256	Column Label		2
15		length	DC	num	8	Column Length		2
16		length	DC1	num	8	Column Length		2
17		memname	DC	char	32	Member Name		2
18		memname	DC1	char	32	Member Name		2
19		name	DC	char	32	Column Name		3
20		name	DC1	char	32	Column Name		3
21	Y	name	_PRODSAVAIL	char	8			3
22		type	DC	char	4	Column Type		2
23		type	DC1	char	4	Column Type		2

Example 4.1.3: Compare Data Values

```
* transpose different data values - apply with caution since may
   not display extra records;
proc compare base=sashelp.class compare=class nosummary;
id name;
run;
```

The partial results show differences in data values.

```
                    The COMPARE Procedure
        Comparison of SASHELP.CLASS with WORK.CLASS
                      (Method=EXACT)

ains 9 observations not in WORK.CLASS.
ariables compare unequal: Age
```

```
             Value Comparison Results for Variables

                   ||      Base    Compare
       Name        ||       Age       Age      Diff.      % Diff
       _____      ||      _____    _____    _____    _____
                   ||
       Alfred      ||    14.0000   10.0000    -4.0000    -28.5714
       Alice       ||    13.0000   10.0000    -3.0000    -23.0769
       Barbara     ||    13.0000   10.0000    -3.0000    -23.0769
```

4.2 NON-MISSING DATASET LABEL

This example accesses metadata from Proc CONTENTS to confirm dataset and variables are non-missing. The first Proc SQL uses the CASE block to check MEMLABEL variable which is the dataset label. The second Proc SQL uses the CASE block to check the LABEL variable value for each variable.

Example 4.2.1: Non-missing Dataset Label

```
proc contents data=sdtm.dm out=dm_contents (rename= (name=
   variable)) noprint position;
run;

proc sql noprint;
create table dc as
select unique 'DM' as domain,
   compbl("SUBJECTID / DM Label") as key_grp_vr length=50
   , memlabel as dc_rslt label="DM Label:" length=200
```

(Continued)

Example 4.2.1 (*Continued*): Non-missing Dataset Label

```
, case when memlabel = '' then 'FAIL: Missing DM Label'
else 'PASS: Non-missing DM Label' end as ctck label="DM Label"
from dm_contents;
quit;

proc sql noprint;
create table dc as
select unique 'DM' as domain,
  compbl("SUBJECTID / DM Label") as key_grp_vr length=50
, label as dc_rslt label="DM Label:" length=200
, case when label = '' then 'FAIL: Missing DM Label'
else 'PASS: Non-missing DM Label' end as ctck label="DM Label"
from dm_contents;
quit;
```

This passes, as both DM dataset and variable labels are all non-missing. The second screen shot shows one row for each variable.

Output

Obs	domain	key_grp_vr	dc_rslt	ctck
1	DM	SUBJECTID / DM Label	Demographics	PASS: Non-missing DM Label

Page Break

Obs	domain	key_grp_vr	dc_rslt	ctck
1	DM	SUBJECTID / DM Label	Actual Arm Code	PASS: Non-missing DM Label
2	DM	SUBJECTID / DM Label	Age	PASS: Non-missing DM Label
3	DM	SUBJECTID / DM Label	Age Units	PASS: Non-missing DM Label
4	DM	SUBJECTID / DM Label	Country	PASS: Non-missing DM Label
5	DM	SUBJECTID / DM Label	Date/Time of Birth	PASS: Non-missing DM Label
6	DM	SUBJECTID / DM Label	Date/Time of Collection	PASS: Non-missing DM Label
7	DM	SUBJECTID / DM Label	Date/Time of Death	PASS: Non-missing DM Label
8	DM	SUBJECTID / DM Label	Date/Time of End of Participation	PASS: Non-missing DM Label
9	DM	SUBJECTID / DM Label	Date/Time of First Study Treatment	PASS: Non-missing DM Label
10	DM	SUBJECTID / DM Label	Date/Time of Informed Consent	PASS: Non-missing DM Label

4.3 NO PERMANENT FORMAT IN DM

The example below accesses metadata from Proc CONTENTS to confirm permanent formats do not exist in SDTMs. Proc SQL uses the CASE block to check the FORMAT variable.

Example 4.3.1: No Permanent Format

```
proc contents data=sdtm.dm out=dm_contents (rename=(name=
    variable)) noprint position;
run;

proc sql noprint;
create table dc as
select unique 'DM' as domain,
  compbl("SUBJECTID / DM Formats") as key_grp_vr length=50
  , memlabel as dc_rslt label="DM Formats:" length=200
  , case when format = '' then 'PASS: Valid Missing DM Formats'
    else 'FAIL: Invalid Non-missing DM Formats' end as ctck
    label="DM Formats"
  from dm_contents;
quit;
```

DC results show that there are no permanent formats in DM.

Output

Obs	domain	key_grp_vr	dc_rslt	ctck
1	DM	SUBJECTID / DM Formats	Demographics	PASS: Valid Missing DM Formats

4.4 DM CORRECT ORDER OF VARIABLES

The example below checks for the correct order and compares the list of variables in DM. Proc CONTENTS is used to access metadata. The first two SELECT statements create macro variables. The third SELECT statement uses a CASE and VERIFY() function to compare the two macro variable lists by name and order. Create macro variable list is created from SDTM specifications containing the variable names. A second macro variable list is created from each domain. Note that both lists are sorted by VARNUM. Then the two lists are compared to each other. Any differences in sort order or variables are then identified. The correct order of SDTM and ADaM variables can be obtained from the specifications and implementation guide. The example below compares DM variables.

Example 4.4.1: Correct Order of Variables

```
proc contents data=sdtm.dm out=dm_contents (rename=
    (name=variable)) noprint position;
run;

proc sql noprint;
select unique name into :sdtm_list separated by ', ' from sashelp.
    vcolumn where libname='SDTM' and memname='DM' order
    by varnum;

* production;
select unique variable into :dc_dm separated by ', ' from dm_
    contents order by varnum;

* pass test;
*select unique variable into :dc_dm separated by ', ' from sdtm
    where dataset='DM' order by order;
quit;
%put &sdtm_list;
%put &dc_dm;

proc sql noprint;
create table dc as
select unique 'DM' as domain,
    compbl("SUBJECTID / DM List") as key_grp_vr length=50
    , "&dc_dm" as dc_rslt label="DM List:" length=200
    , "&sdtm_list" as sdtm_rslt label="SDTM DM List:" length=200
    , case when verify(trim("&dc_dm"), "&sdtm_list") then 'FAIL:
        Invalid DM List'
    else 'PASS: Valid DM List' end as ctck label="DM List"
    from sdtm.dm;
quit;
```

The partial DC revels that there are no difference in the sort order or list of DM variables. Note that this check works well to confirm all required variables exist.

Output

Obs	domain	key_grp_vr	dc_rslt		sdtm_rs
					STUDYI
					RFSTDT
					RFXENC
					DTHDTC
					AGEU, S
				STUDYID, DOMAIN, USUBJID, SUBJID, RFSTDTC, RFENDTC, RFXSTDTC, RFXENDTC, RFICDTC, RFPENDTC, DTHDTC, DTHFL, SITEID, BRTHDTC,	ACTARM
1	DM	SUBJECTID / DM List	AGE, AGEU, SEX, RACE, ETHNIC, ARMCD, ARM, ACTARMCD, ACTARM, COUNTRY, DMDTC, D		D

4.5 VARIABLE LENGTH IS MAXIMUM OF VALUES OR 200

Initially in DDTs, SDTM character variables may be set to 200 to prevent truncation. However, by submission time, the character variables must be reset to the actual maximum length to conserve space. The example below determines the maximum variable length by domain and variable based on all patient records. With this metadata information, datasets are re-created with LENGTH statements for each character variable before applying the SET statement.

The MAXLEN temporary dataset contains the name of each dataset that contains character variables, the names of the character variables and the maximum length of the three work datasets AA, AB and AC. The DATA _ NULL_ step below creates a DATA step for each dataset in the metadata. In addition, it issues a LENGTH statement for each character variable in that dataset setting the length to the maximum found in any dataset. This grouping is done with similar variables because of Proc SQL's GROUP BY NAME. The code is written directly to the macro processor with the CALL EXECUTE() statements so that each domain DATA step will run after the DATA _NULL_ step completes. The FIRST.DSNAME statement creates the DATA statement, then each record creates the LENGTH statement for each variable and finally the LAST.DSNAME statement creates the SET and RUN statements. Notice that the CAT() function is used to concatenate SAS statements together. This will readjust each domain with the maximum character variable lengths. You can then compare the updated and original SDTMs using the metadata comparison in Example 4.5.1.

Example 4.5.1: Variables Length Is Max Values

```
data aa;
a='123456789';
b='12345';
c='1234567890123456';
```

(Continued)

Example 4.5.1 (*Continued*): Variables Length Is Max Values

```
d='123456789012345678901234567890';
e='12345678901234567890';
f='1';
run;

data ab;
a='123456789';
b='12345';
c='1234567890123456';
d='12345678901234567890';
e='123456789012345678901234567890';
g='1';
run;

data ac;
a='123456789';
b='12345678901234567890';
c='1234567890123456';
d='123456789012345678901234567890';
e='12345';
h='1';
run;

%let targetlib=work;
%let workingtbl=maxlen;

proc sql;
create table &workingtbl. as
select memname as dsname, name as varnam, max(length)as
   varlen from dictionary.columns
where libname=upcase("&targetlib") and type='char' group by
   name order by memname, name;
quit;

data _null_;
set &workingtbl. end=done;
by dsname;
```

(*Continued*)

Example 4.5.1 (*Continued*): Variables Length Is Max Values

```
if first.dsname then do;
  call execute(cat('data ', "&targetlib.." || trim(dsname),';'));
end;
call execute(cat('length ', trim(varnam), ' $',varlen,';'));
if last.dsname then do;
  call execute(cat('set ', "&targetlib.." || trim(dsname),'; run;'));
end;
run;
```

The output shows the syntax dynamically created for the same max length dataset in AA and AB. Note that the macro first determined the max length across all three datasets for the same variable names. The AA dataset below shows no truncation in data values.

Output

```
NOTE: CALL EXECUTE generated line.
1             + data work.AA;
2             + length a $9;
3             + length b $20;
4             + length c $16;
5             + length d $30;
6             + length e $30;
7             + length f $1;
8             + set work.AA; run;

NOTE: There were 1 observations read from the data set WORK.AA.
NOTE: The data set WORK.AA has 1 observations and 6 variables.
NOTE: DATA statement used (Total process time):
      real time           0.00 seconds
      cpu time            0.00 seconds


9             + data work.AB;
10            + length a $9;
11            + length b $20;
12            + length c $16;
13            + length d $30;
14            + length e $30;
15            + length g $1;
16            + set work.AB; run;

NOTE: There were 1 observations read from the data set WORK.AB.
NOTE: The data set WORK.AB has 1 observations and 6 variables.
```

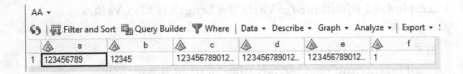

The example below confirms all XXTEST variable name lengths, and data lengths are no longer than 40. Proc SQL uses VCOLUMN metadata on NAME and LENGTH.

Example 4.5.2: XXTEST Variables Length Is Less than or Equal to 40

```
proc sql;
create table dc as
select memname, name, length
from sashelp.vcolumn where libname eq 'SDTM' and index(name,
   'TEST') > 0 and (length(name) gt 40 or length gt 40);
quit;
```

For the checks that fail, the output shows SDTM and variable names and their lengths.

Output

Obs	memname	name	length
1	IE	IETEST	159
2	TE	TESTRL	63
3	TI	IETEST	197

SUMMARY

This chapter provides examples of CDISC specification compliance checks. CDISC specification compliance checks are important first tests to pass in the review process. The FDA first checks the submission metadata to assure required components exist before even reading the data in their system. If the metadata is incomplete or incorrect based on the define.xml, the FDA may immediately reject the submission.

CHAPTER 5

CDISC Data Compliance Checks

INTRODUCTION

The difference between SDTM and ADaM Data checks and CDISC Data Compliance checks is that now the focus is on data content and CDISC structure rules. CDISC data compliance checks are broken down into SDTM and ADaM consistency checks. SDTM examples of these checks include consistency between AENUM and CMAENUM and between RELREC and SDTMs. ADaM checks include valid DTYPE values and consistency between the analysis visit window and protocol. The CDISC data compliance checks must pass through Pinnacle 21 checks.

5.1 SDTM CONSISTENCY

Checks below are examples from one domain. When needed, it is recommended to create macros to loop through each domain.

5.1.1 AENUM and CENUM

When collected on the case report forms, AE and CM will be linked by AENUM and CMAENUM to adverse events with conmeds. Creating this link between AE and CM can be challenging. The example below searches for AENUM within a collection of numbers in CMAENUM. The code identifies matched values greater than 0. The INDEXW() function searches for AENUM, as is, within CMAENUM.

Example 5.1.1.1: AENUM and CENUM

```
proc sql;
create table cm_ae as
select unique a.usubjid, a.cmaenum, b.aenum, a.cmtrt, b.aedecod
from adcm as a full join adae as b on a.usubjid=b.usubjid
  where cmstdy > 0 and indexw(cmaenum, aenum, ' ,')
    > 0 and cmiss(cmaenum, aenum)= 0;
quit;
```

The partial results below link CM and AE by matching AENUM. Both CMTRT and AEDECOD can be reviewed and confirmed. We can see that AENUM values are contained within CMAENUM values.

Output

Obs	USUBJID	CMAENUM	AENUM	CMTRT	AEDECOD
1	▮▮▮-101-001-004	12,13	12	ACETAMINOPHEN TAB	Pain
2	▮▮▮-101-001-004	48,49,50,51,52	48	NEUPOGEN IV	White blood cell count decreased

5.1.2 AE.AESEQ and SUPPAE.IDVARVAL

For SUPPXX datasets to be valid, they must all be linked back to their corresponding XX domain. The XXSEQ and IDVARVAL need to be in sync by USUBJID. The example below creates a key variable based on using CATX() to concatenating USUBJID and IDVARVAL from SUPPAE and compares that to concatenating USUBJID and AESEQ from AE. The DCB dataset will contain any mismatches. If DCB has zero observations, then there are no mismatches.

Example 5.1.2.1: AE.AESEQ and SUPPAE.IDVARVAL

```
proc sql number;
create table dca as
 select unique catx(' ', usubjid, idvarval) as suppkey
from suppae;

 create table dcb as
 select *
from dca where suppkey not in (select unique catx(' ', usubjid,
    aeseq) from ae);
quit;
```

The example below is a simple method to create EXSEQ and compare with production EXSEQ. EXSEQ is created from the BY group USUBJID and EXSTDTC.

Example 5.1.2.2: Source and qc EXSEQ

```
proc sort data=ex;
by usubjid exstdtc;
run;

data ex1;
set ex;
by usubjid exstdtc;

if first.usubjid then exseq=1;
 else exseq + 1;
run;

proc compare data=ex compare=ex1;
var exseq;
id usubjid;
run;
```

The results are consistent between source and qc EXSEQ since no unequal values are displayed in Proc COMPARE.

Output

```
NOTE: No unequal values were found. All values compared are exactly equal.
```

5.1.3 Orphan Records in SUPPXX

Since QVAL values in SUPPXX can be incorrectly created without any reference to XX, it is important to confirm no orphan records exist in SUPPXX. The example below checks for orphan records in SUPPDM. This can be repeated for all other SUPPXX.

Example 5.1.3.1: Orphan Records in SUPPXX

```
proc transpose data=suppdm out=suppdm1 (drop = _name_ _label_);
by usubjid;
var qval;
id qnam;
idlabel qlabel;
run;
proc print; run;

proc sort data=suppdm1;
  by usubjid;
run;

data dm1;
  merge dm suppdm1;
  by usubjid;
run;

* proc compare with adsl for suppdm variables kept;
proc compare data=adsl compare=dm1;
var phase;
id usubjid;
run;
```

The dataset below is the transposition of SUPPDM with the variables as column. Next, Proc COMPARE compares the SUPPDM with those from ADSL. Any unequal values indicate potential orphan records in SUPPDM.

Output

Obs		AGEENRL	COHRTPH2	PHASE	COHRTPH1	RACEOTH
1		56	Cohort 1 (DLBCL)	Phase2		
2		58	Cohort 2 (PMBCL/TFL)	Phase2		
3		62	Cohort 1 (DLBCL)	Phase2		
4		56	Cohort 1 (DLBCL)	Phase2		
5		60	Cohort 3	Phase2		
6		69	Cohort 3	Phase2		
7		59		Phase1	A1	
8		53		Phase1	A1	
9		69		Phase1	A1	
10		69		Phase1	A1	

```
Total Number of Values which Compare Unequal: 26.
```

5.1.4 DOMAIN Variable and Name

The example below confirms DOMAIN equals the domain name. A macro can be written to loop through each domain. As an alternative, the DSNAME() metadata function with the dataset ID can be used to return the domain name.

Example 5.1.4.1: DOMAIN Variable and Name

```
proc sql;
create table dc as
select unique 'DM' as domain,
  compbl("SUBJECTID / Domain") as key_grp_vr length=50
, case when domain ^= "DM" then 'FAIL: Invalid Domain'
  else 'PASS: Valid Domain' end as ctck label="Domain Codelist"
  from dm;
quit;
```

DC results are consistent between DOMAIN and domain name.

Output

Obs	domain	key_grp_vr	ctck
1	DM	SUBJECTID / Domain	PASS: Valid Domain

5.1.5 Required SDTM Domains (TA, DM, EX and DS) Do Not Exist

In the final submission, key SDTMs such as TA, DM, EX and DS need to be included. The example below is one method to confirm these required SDTMs. Proc FORMAT creates $SDTM and $ADAM formats, which group SDTMs and ADaMs. $SDTM format is applied to MEMNAME to display required and other categories. Additional SDTMs can be added to the required list.

Example 5.1.5.1: Required SDTM Domains

```
proc format;
value $sdtm 'TA', 'DM', 'EX', 'DS' = 'Four Required SDTMs'
other = 'Other SDTMs';
value $adam 'ADSL' = 'ADSL Required'
other = 'Other ADaMs';
run;

* Must have 4 in Four Required SDTMs column;
proc tabulate data=sashelp.vtable missing;
class memname;
tables memname / printmiss;
format memname $sdtm.;
where libname in ('SDTM');
run;

* SDTM record counts;
proc sql;
  create table dc as
  select libname, memname, nobs from dictionary.tables where
    libname in ('SDTM') and memname in ('TA', 'DM', 'EX', 'DS');
quit;
```

The results show the four required SDTMs exist. The second screen shows the number of observations for required SDTMs. From this, we can confirm required SDTMs exist.

Output

Member Name	
Other SDTMs	Four Required SDTMs
N	N
61	4

Page Break

Obs	libname	memname	nobs
1	SDTM	DM	187
2	SDTM	DS	1626
3	SDTM	EX	1143
4	SDTM	TA	14

5.1.6 Required ADaMs (ADSL) Do Not Exist

The example below is the corresponding required ADaMs check for ADSL. $ADAM format is applied to MEMNAME to display required and other categories. Other ADaMs can be added to the required list.

Example 5.1.6.1: Required ADaMs

```
* Repeat for required ADaMs do not exit exist - ADSL;
proc tabulate data=sashelp.vtable missing;
class memname;
tables memname / printmiss;
format memname $adam.;
where libname in ('ADAM');
run;

* ADaM record counts;
proc sql;
  create table dc as
  select libname, memname, nobs from dictionary.tables where
    libname in ('ADAM') and memname in ('ADSL');
quit;
```

The results show ADSL exists. The second screenshot shows the number of observations in ADSL.

Output

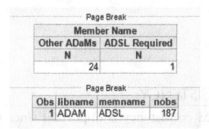

Member Name	
Other ADaMs N	ADSL Required N
24	1

Obs	libname	memname	nobs
1	ADAM	ADSL	187

5.1.7 SE Start and End Dates Sequence Requirement

The example below checks for out of sequence of start and end dates in SE. By using the LAG() function, we can have access to the previous record data from the current record. This allows us to compare start and end dates across sequential records.

Example 5.1.7.1: SE Start and End Dates

```
proc sort data=sdtm.se out= se;
by usubjid seseq element sestdtc seendtc;
run;

data dc;
length lag_sestdtc lag_seendtc $16.;
set se;
 by usubjid seseq element sestdtc seendtc;

if first.usubjid then do; lag_sestdtc="; lag_seendtc = "; end;
lag_sestdtc = lag(sestdtc);
lag_seendtc = lag(seendtc);

if ^first.usubjid and sestdtc ^= lag_seendtc then flag='Y';
 else if ^first.usubjid and sestdtc < lag_sstndtc then flag='Y';
 else if ^first.usubjid and seendtc < lag_seendtc then flag='Y';
 else if sestdtc > seendtc then flag='Y';
 else flag=";
run;
```

The partial results below show SE start dates after end dates. These are obvious data errors that need to be resolved.

Output

eendtc	STUDYID	DOMAIN	USUBJID	SESEQ	ETCD	ELEMENT	SESTDTC	SEENDTC	TAETORD	SEUPDES	SESTDY	SEENDY	flag	lag_sstndtc
29-03	-101	SE	-101-002-003	6	LFU	Long Term Follow-up	2015-09-03	2015-08-26	7		94	86	Y	
03-30	-101	SE	-101-003-007	6	LFU	Long Term Follow-up	2016-03-30	2015-11-17	7		90	-44	Y	
06-16	-101	SE	-101-005-003	6	LFU	Long Term Follow-up	2016-06-16	2016-04-18	7		79	20	Y	

5.2 ADaM CONSISTENCY

Checking for ADaM consistency is important since there is more data management tasks in creating ADaM compared to SDTMs. In ADaMs, records can be derived and added by USUBJID. The example below checks derived DTYPE records. When needed, it is recommended to create macros to loop through each ADaM.

The example below creates a new DTYPE='Average' by USUBJID and PARAMCD. Along with creating this record is the correct placement of the new record so that the record relates to the individual records. Proc SQL uses an OUTER UNION CORR to append the average records by USUBJID, PARAMCD and AVISITN. The average records are created from the subquery, which groups by USUBJID and PARAMCD. The technique can be used for other summary functions, such as MIN() or MAX() instead of AVG().

Example 5.2.1.1: Valid DTYPE

```
proc sql;
create table dc as select a.usubjid, a.avisitn, a.paramcd, a.aval
from adbmk as a
outer union corr
( select "Average" as dtype ,
         round(avg(aval), .01) as ck_aval,
         usubjid, paramcd
  from adbmk (where=(avisitn > .)) as b
  group by usubjid, paramcd )
order by usubjid, paramcd, avisitn;
quit;
```

The partial results below show the DTYPE='Average' record is grouped with the USUBJID records that were used to create the average values from AVAL. Now the CK_AVAL variable can be checked with the ADaM average value by USUBJID and PARAMCD. It is a CDISC requirement to keep average records next to the corresponding USUBJID and PARAMCD records when FDA reviews the dataset. This sort order is easier to review than creating all average records toward the end of the ADaM. As expected, DTYPE is missing for all other records.

Output

Obs	USUBJID	AVISITN	PARAMCD	AVAL	dtype	ck_aval
1	101-001-004	.	AMYLOIDA	.	Average	54485728.64
2	101-001-004	.	AMYLOIDA	2728599.7		.
3	101-001-004	-5	AMYLOIDA	18722894.0		.
4	101-001-004	0	AMYLOIDA	19282528.0		.
5	101-001-004	1	AMYLOIDA	5968536.8		.
6	101-001-004	3	AMYLOIDA	126782218.9		.
7	101-001-004	5	AMYLOIDA	296058363.3		.
8	101-001-004	7	AMYLOIDA	2698487.0		.
9	101-001-004	14	AMYLOIDA	417638.7		.
10	101-001-004	28	AMYLOIDA	1536971.3		.
11	101-001-004	90	AMYLOIDA	18903919.8		.

SUMMARY

This chapter provides examples of CDISC data compliance level checks. While initially it may not be obvious, the FDA review process is greatly improved by having submissions that meet all compliance requirements. Organizations must realize that FDA submissions service multiple customers, who view the data and information differently. Organizations have a better chance or speedier approval when all requirements are satisfied.

CHAPTER 6

Protocol Compliance Checks

INTRODUCTION

In general, the SAP defines protocol compliance requirements for both safety and efficacy data. Protocol compliance checks include missing USUBID, invalid lab baseline values and discrepancies in exposure and/or daily dose data. Each study can have customized checks to assure protocol compliance.

6.1 USUBJID MISSING IN DM/ADSL

In some cases, USUBJID is missing in DM or ADSL but exists in other SDTMs or ADaMs. This can happen from extra USUBJID raw data. It is important to monitor this since all USUBJID must exist in DM and ADSL. The SAS program below shows two examples each with datasets, DCA and DCB. Both examples confirm all USUBJID in ADAE, but the second example will fail for testing purposes. Proc SQL uses LEFT JOIN and subqueries since the list of USUBJID must be extracted from ADSL. The GOOD_VALUE will be set to 1 for matched USUBJID, so any records with missing GOOD_VALUE will be extra USUBJID in ADAE. The second example shows a FAILed USUBJID check. DCA identifies which records fail the check, and DCB identifies the overall check.

Example 6.1.1: USUBJID Missing in DM/ADSL

```
proc sql;
create table dca as
   select unique a.usubjid, b.good_value from adae as a
   left join
   (select usubjid, count(usubjid) as good_value label='USUBJID
      exists in ADSL' from adsl) as b on a.usubjid = b.usubjid;

create table dcb as
select unique 'ADAE' as domain,
   compbl("USUBJID / ADSL Subset") as key_grp_vr length=50
   , case when nmiss(good_value) >= 1 then 'FAIL: At least one
      USUBJID Not in ADSL'
   else 'PASS: All USUBJID in ADSL' end as dc_rslt label="Data
      Check Results For:" length=75
   from dca;
quit;

* Condition test - should not pass test with test case for first pt;
data adsl1;
set adsl;
if _n_ = 1 then delete;
run;

* must use subquery since different datasets, Should pass test
since adae is subset of adsl;
proc sql;
create table dca as
   select a.usubjid, b.good_value from adae as a
   left join
   (select usubjid, count(usubjid) as good_value label='USUBJID
      exists in ADSL' from adsl1) as b on a.usubjid = b.usubjid;

create table dcb as
select unique 'ADAE' as domain,
```

Example 6.1.1 (*Continued*): USUBJID Missing in DM/ADSL

```
compbl("USUBJID / ADSL Subset") as key_grp_vr length=50
, case when nmiss(good_value) >= 1 then 'FAIL: At least one
  USUBJID Not in ADSL'
else 'PASS: All USUBJID in ADSL' end as dc_rslt label="Data
  Check Results For:" length=75
from dca;
quit;
```

The first example shows PASS for all ADAE USUBJIDs in ADSL. The second example identifies USUBJID in ADAE but not in ADSL, since in this example the first USUBJID was deleted.

Output

Obs	domain	key_grp_vr	dc_rslt
1	ADAE	USUBJID / ADSL Subset	PASS: All USUBJID in ADSL

--- Page Break ---

Obs	domain	key_grp_vr	dc_rslt
1	ADAE	USUBJID / ADSL Subset	FAIL: At least one USUBJID Not in ADSL

6.2 MISSING EXPOSURE RECORD IN EX FOR DM USUBJID

In general, it is expected that all USUBJID in DM have at least one exposure record in EX unless the USUBJID is a screen failure or ended study after randomization but before first dose. For patients randomized to treatment dose, it is important to monitor corresponding exposure records to assure protocol compliance administration requirements. One potential reason for failing this check is maybe due to delays in entering the data in the system. This example is similar to the previous example, except that conditions are applied to DM to account for unexpected exposure records. Within Proc SQL, dataset options are still valid to subset the dataset for example. Once SCRNFAIL and NOTASSGN records are excluded from DM, all remaining USUBJID can be cross-checked with EX. When USUBJID exists in DM but not in EX, it indicates a missing exposure record in EX. DCA identifies which records fail, and DCB identifies the overall check. This example can be repeated for DS.

Example 6.2.1: Missing Exposure Record Using Method 1

```
proc sql;
create table dca as
  select unique a.usubjid, actarmcd, b.good_value from dm
    (where=(actarmcd ^in ('SCRNFAIL' 'NOTASSGN'))) as a

  left join
  (select usubjid, count(usubjid) as good_value label='USUBJID
    exists in DM' from ex) as b on a.usubjid = b.usubjid;

create table dcb as
select unique 'EX' as domain,
  compbl("SUBJECTID / DM Subset") as key_grp_vr length=50
  , case when nmiss(good_value) >= 1 then 'FAIL: At least one
    USUBJID Not in DM'
  else 'PASS: All USUBJID in DM' end as dc_rslt label="Data
    Check Results For:" length=75
  from dca;
quit;
```

The results show all USUBJIDs in DM are in EX.

Output

Obs	domain	key_grp_vr	dc_rslt
1	EX	SUBJECTID / DM Subset	PASS: All USUBJID in DM

Example 6.2.2: Missing Exposure Record Using Method 2

As an alternative to the previous example, the SAS programs below identify USUBJID not in DM using the NOT IN operator and EXCEPT option. The first example checks EX, and the second example checks AE. Both methods will give consistent results in DC. Note that this method requires only selecting USUBJID instead of all other variables since only USUBJID values are compared.

```
* Alternative method 1 selects only USUBJID NOT in DM;
proc sql;
create table dc as
select usubjid from dm where usubjid not in (select distinct
    usubjid from ex);
quit;

* Alternative method 2 selects only USUBJID NOT in DM;
proc sql;
create table dc as
select unique usubjid from DM
 except
select unique usubjid from AE;
quit;
```

Example 6.2.3: Missing Exposure Record Using Method 3

As a final alternative to the previous example, the SAS program below shows how to identify NAME not in CLASS dataset. The GOOD_LST dataset is created with only the required NAMES. In this example, only John is kept in GOOD_LST. The GOOD_LST can then be used as a lookup table for CLASS dataset.

```
* Alternative method 3 selects only SUBJECTID records NOT in
DM;
* Create test dataset;
data good_lst;
set sashelp.class;
if name='John';
run;

proc sql;
create table dc as
select *, 'FAIL: USUBJID Not in DM' as bad_value  from sashelp.class
where name not in (select unique name from good_lst);
quit;
```

All NAMEs in CLASS FAIL since they do not equal John.

Output

Obs	Name	Sex	Age	Height	Weight	bad_value
1	Alfred	M	14	69.0	112.5	FAIL: USUBJID Not in DM
2	Alice	F	13	56.5	84.0	FAIL: USUBJID Not in DM
3	Barbara	F	13	65.3	98.0	FAIL: USUBJID Not in DM
4	Carol	F	14	62.8	102.5	FAIL: USUBJID Not in DM
5	Henry	M	14	63.5	102.5	FAIL: USUBJID Not in DM
6	James	M	12	57.3	83.0	FAIL: USUBJID Not in DM
7	Jane	F	12	59.8	84.5	FAIL: USUBJID Not in DM
8	Janet	F	15	62.5	112.5	FAIL: USUBJID Not in DM
9	Jeffrey	M	13	62.5	84.0	FAIL: USUBJID Not in DM
10	Joyce	F	11	51.3	50.5	FAIL: USUBJID Not in DM
11	Judy	F	14	64.3	90.0	FAIL: USUBJID Not in DM
12	Louise	F	12	56.3	77.0	FAIL: USUBJID Not in DM
13	Mary	F	15	66.5	112.0	FAIL: USUBJID Not in DM
14	Philip	M	16	72.0	150.0	FAIL: USUBJID Not in DM
15	Robert	M	12	64.8	128.0	FAIL: USUBJID Not in DM
16	Ronald	M	15	67.0	133.0	FAIL: USUBJID Not in DM
17	Thomas	M	11	57.5	85.0	FAIL: USUBJID Not in DM
18	William	M	15	66.5	112.0	FAIL: USUBJID Not in DM

6.3 LAB DATA BASELINE

The determination of baseline lab data is a critical for primary or secondary endpoint analysis. The examples below confirm baseline flag records.

6.3.1 Incorrect ADBLFL Baseline Flag Record

The baseline measure is often identified as the last lab measurement before dose administration. In general, baseline flags are derived in ADaMs in a BDS structure. This check confirms correct baseline lab values. DCA creates GOOD_VALUE using Proc SQL's LEFT JOIN and subquery with WHERE condition to filter records, HAVING condition to filter by summary function and GROUP BY. DCB has CASE block with condition to confirm LBBLFL and GOOD_VALUE.

Example 6.3.1: Incorrect ADBLFL Baseline Flag Record

```
proc sql;
create table dca as
   select a.usubjid, a.lbtestcd, a.lbblfl, a.lbdy, a.lbstresn, b.good_value
     from sdtm.lbcy as a
   left join
```

(*Continued*)

Example 6.3.1 (*Continued*): Incorrect ADBLFL Baseline Flag Record

```
(select usubjid, lbtestcd, lbdy as good_value label='Baseline
  Record' from sdtm.lbcy
where lbdy < 0 group by usubjid, lbtestcd having lbdy=max(lbdy))
  as b on a.usubjid = b.usubjid and a.lbtestcd=b.lbtestcd;

create table dcb as
select unique 'LB' as domain,
  compbl("USUBJID / lbblfl Subset") as key_grp_vr length=50
  , case when lbblfl='Y' and ^(lbdy=good_value) then 'FAIL: At least
    one Baseline is Not correct'
  else 'PASS: All Baselines are correct' end as dc_rslt label="Data
    Check Results For:" length=75
  from dca;
quit;

proc sort data=dca;
by usubjid lbtestcd lbdy;
run;
proc print data=dcb; run;
```

Since DCB shows both PASS and FAIL, that means there are baseline flags that are correct and at least one baseline flag that is incorrect. DCA identifies which patient lab tests fail the baseline flag check.

Output

Obs	domain	key_grp_vr	dc_rslt
1	LB	USUBJID / lbblfl Subset	FAIL: At least one Baseline is Not correct
2	LB	USUBJID / lbblfl Subset	PASS: All Baselines are correct

6.3.2 No Baseline Result for VS, LB, EG, DA

Another case is the possibility of missing baseline results, which can be caused by missing values or unexpected raw data. A separate check is performed to minimize the number of missing baseline results. The three examples below are variations of checking baseline results. DCA identifies which records fail, and DCB identifies the overall check.

Example 6.3.2: No Baseline Results

```
* Case 1;
proc sql;
create table dca as
  select a.usubjid, a.lbtestcd, a.lbblfl, a.lbdy, a.lbstresn, b.good_value
    from lb as a
  left join
  (select usubjid, lbtestcd, lbdy as good_value label='Baseline
    Record' from lb
  where lbdy < 0 group by usubjid, lbtestcd having lbdy=
  max(lbdy)) as b on a.usubjid = b.usubjid and a.lbtestcd=b.
  lbtestcd;

create table dcb as
select unique 'LB' as domain,
  compbl("USUBJID / lbblfl Subset") as key_grp_vr length=50
  , case when lbblfl='Y' and ^(lbdy=good_value) then 'FAIL:
    At least one Baseline is Not correct'
  else 'PASS: All Baselines are correct' end as dc_rslt label="Data
    Check Results For:" length=75
  from dca;
quit;
proc sort data=dca;
by usubjid lbtestcd lbdy;
run;

* Case 2;
proc sql;
create table dca as
  select a.usubjid, a.lbtestcd, a.lbblfl, a.visit, a.lbstresn, b.good_
    value from lb as a
  left join
  (select usubjid, lbtestcd, 1 as good_value label='Baseline
    Subset' from lb where lbblfl='Y' group by usubjid, lbtestcd)
    as b on a.usubjid = b.usubjid and a.lbtestcd=b.lbtestcd;
```

(Continued)

Example 6.3.2 (*Continued*): No Baseline Results

```
create table dcb as
select unique 'LB' as domain,
  compbl("USUBJID / lbblfl Subset") as key_grp_vr length=50
  , case when nmiss(good_value) >= 1 then 'FAIL: At least one
    subject Without Baseline'
  else 'PASS: All subjects with Baseline' end as dc_rslt label="Data
    Check Results For:" length=75
  from dca;
quit;


* Case 3;
* Condition test - should pass test with all pts with baseline;
data lb1;
set lb;
if usubjid ^='101-001-004' then delete;
run;

proc sql;
create table dca as
  select a.usubjid, a.lbtestcd, b.good_value from lb1 as a
  left join
  (select usubjid, lbtestcd, 1 as good_value label='Baseline
    Subset' from lb1 where lbblfl='Y' group by usubjid,
    lbtestcd) as b on a.usubjid = b.usubjid and a.lbtestcd=b.lbtestcd;

create table dcb as
select unique 'LB' as domain,
  compbl("USUBJID / lbblfl Subset") as key_grp_vr length=50
  , case when nmiss(good_value) >= 1 then 'FAIL: At least one
    subject Without Baseline'
  else 'PASS: All subjects with Baseline' end as dc_rslt label="Data
    Check Results For:" length=75
  from dca;
quit;
```

The first case result PASSed the check for correct baselines. The second case result FAILed the check with at least one USUBJID without a baseline flag. Finally, the third case result PASSed the check for correct baselines.

Output

Obs	domain	key_grp_vr	dc_rslt
1	LB	USUBJID / lbblfl Subset	PASS: All Baselines are correct

———————————————— Page Break ————————————————

Obs	domain	key_grp_vr	dc_rslt
1	LB	USUBJID / lbblfl Subset	FAIL: At least one subject Without Baseline

———————————————— Page Break ————————————————

Obs	domain	key_grp_vr	dc_rslt
1	LB	USUBJID / lbblfl Subset	PASS: All subjects with Baseline

6.4 DISPOSITION TREE CHECK – ONE-PROC AWAY

One of the advantages of ADaMs is having the power of one-Proc away. This means that SAS procedures can be directly applied to ADaMs to get summarized information, such as descriptive statistics and/or frequency counts. The disposition tree check is useful to track all patients from study entry to study completion as shown in Figure A.3. Proc FREQ with LIST options provides frequency counts instead of the standard grid format. The MISSING option includes missing values.

Example 6.4.1: Disposition Tree

```
proc freq data=DS;
tables DSSEQ*DSCAT*DSTERM/list missing;
run;

*** Get All Randomized Subjects Status;
proc sort data = DS (where=(usubjid ne ' ' and dsscat ne ' '))
out = ds (keep=usubjid dscat dsscat dsstdtc);
by usubjid dscat dsscat dsstdtc;
run;
```

(Continued)

Example 6.4.1 (*Continued*): Disposition Tree

```
*** Separate discontinued and completed status for both base
    and extension phases;
data discon comp;
set ds;
if dsscat eq 'DISCONTINUED' then output discon;
else if dsscat eq 'COMPLETED' then output comp;
run;

*** If discontinuation date is before the completion date, it is a
    data issue;
data bad_discon_before_comp;
merge discon(in=dd rename=(dsstdtc=dis_dt) drop=dscat dss-
    cat) comp(in=cc);
by usubjid;
if dd and cc and (dis_dt < dsstdtc);
run;
```

The partial results display a combination of DSCAT and DSTERM frequency counts so that patient disposition can be confirmed as far as the number still in study or terminated.

Output

DSSEQ	DSCAT	DSTERM	Frequency	Percent	Cumulative Frequency	Cumulative Percent
1	PROTOCOL MILESTONE	STUDY INFORMED CONSENT OBTAINED	187	11.50	187	11.50
2	DISPOSITION EVENT	SCREEN FAILURE	11	0.68	198	12.18
2	PROTOCOL MILESTONE	STUDY INFORMED CONSENT OBTAINED	8	0.49	206	12.67
2	PROTOCOL MILESTONE	SUBJECT ENROLLED	74	4.55	280	17.22
2	PROTOCOL MILESTONE	TUMOR BIOPSY INFORMED CONSENT OBTAINED	94	5.78	374	23.00
3	DISPOSITION EVENT	ADVERSE EVENT	4	0.25	378	23.25
3	DISPOSITION EVENT	COMPLETED TREATMENT	21	1.29	399	24.54
3	DISPOSITION EVENT	DEATH	1	0.06	400	24.60
3	DISPOSITION EVENT	PRODUCT NOT AVAILABLE	1	0.06	401	24.66
3	DISPOSITION EVENT	SCREEN FAILURE	15	0.92	416	25.58
3	PROTOCOL MILESTONE	STUDY INFORMED CONSENT OBTAINED	55	3.38	471	28.97
3	PROTOCOL MILESTONE	SUBJECT ENROLLED	78	4.80	549	33.76
3	PROTOCOL MILESTONE	TUMOR BIOPSY INFORMED CONSENT OBTAINED	1	0.06	550	33.83

SUMMARY

This chapter provides examples of protocol compliance checks. In the final FDA submission, strict protocol compliance must be validated. Often, there are many protocol amendments that need confirmation and adjustments based on more exploratory analysis.

CHAPTER 7

Codelist Dictionary Compliance Checks

INTRODUCTION

Codelist dictionary compliance checks are the heart of unit-level checks, which is one of the five channels of the CDISC compliance issues chart in Figure 1.4. Since all raw data is now standardized to controlled terminology, there are many opportunities for cross-checking clinical data with codelist dictionary tables. In addition, the define.xml file must have a correct and updated codelist section. Codelist dictionaries can be created for both SDTMs and ADaMs. The first example below automatically creates a codelist dictionary across all SDTMs, and the second example compares codelist dictionaries from SDTMs and define.xml specifications. Both examples are essential to meet CDISC compliance. Codelist dictionary compliance checks are consistent with Pinnacle 21's controlled terminology checks. Keep in mind that versions of SDTM and ADaM controlled terminology dictionaries need to be tracked. Note that without an automated process to create codelist dictionaries, the alternative method of applying Proc FREQ on all categorical variables is very time consuming.

See the following define.xml specification mindmaps in the appendix to have a better understanding of domain sheets and compliance rules for creating define.xml files.

- Define XML Spec Domain Sheets
- Define XML Spec Domain Sheet: Variable Columns
- Define XML Spec Domain Sheet: Origin Column
- Define XML Spec Codelist Columns

7.1 CODELIST, VALUE-LEVEL CHECKS AND LOOKUP TABLES

The application and management of ADaM codelists and lookup tables are essential to keep metadata in sync with codelist dictionary versions.

The example below creates a dictionary Excel file of all ADaM codelists as columns. Since ADaMs contain both continuous and categorical variables, additional code is included to exclude unwanted ADaMs or continuous variables for which codelists do not make sense, else the default is to include all ADaMs and variables. This is useful to see all unique values across all ADaMs. This allows cross-referencing ADaM codelists with the controlled terminology. The code below can also be applied to create SDTM codelist dictionaries. Note that this example contains advanced macro programming to create and loop through records, dynamically creating macro calls for each ADaM and variable. Each intermediate dataset is then merged together in the same correct order so that codelists are grouped by ADaMs and variable order. Once all of the macro calls are created in a separate file, the file is included in the program and executed.

Example 7.1.1: ADaM Codelist Dictionary

```
* Automatically create dataset codelist Excel file;
libname dsn '\\analysis\data\adam' access=readonly;

* for codelist differences make macro call and copy codelist from
    Excel file;
%MACRO CODEV(libn, dsn, varn, runnum=2)/minoperator;

%if &varn=LBCAT or &varn=LBNAM or &varn=LBSCAT or
    &varn=LBSTAT or &varn=LBTEST or &varn=LBTESTCD
    %then %do;
```

(*Continued*)

Example 7.1.1 (*Continued*): ADaM Codelist Dictionary

```
ods output OneWayFreqs=&dsn._&varn(rename =(&varn
    = &dsn._&varn) keep = &varn);
proc freq data=&libn..&dsn;
  tables &varn/nocol norow nocum nopercent;
run;
%end;
%else %do;
ods output OneWayFreqs=&varn(keep = &varn);
proc freq data=&libn..&dsn;
  tables &varn/nocol norow nocum nopercent;
run;
%end;

* account for same variables across domains;
%if &runnum=1 %then %do;
data codev;
set &varn;
run;
%end;
%else %if &runnum=2 and &varn^=LBCAT and
    &varn^=LBNAM and &varn^=LBSCAT and &varn^=LBSTAT
    and &varn^=LBTEST and &varn^=LBTESTCD  %then %do;
data codev;
merge codev &varn;
run;
%end;
%else %if &runnum=2 and &varn=LBCAT or &varn=LBNAM
    or &varn=LBSCAT or &varn=LBSTAT or &varn=LBTEST or
    &varn=LBTESTCD %then %do;
data codev;
merge codev &dsn._&varn;
run;
%end;
%mend codev;
```

(*Continued*)

Example 7.1.1 (*Continued*): ADaM Codelist Dictionary

```
%*CODEV(dsn, adsl, siteid , runnum=1);
%*CODEV(dsn, adsl, aphase );

* create metadata of dataset and variable names;
* delete all dates, num vars, etc;
* and memname in ('DM' 'AE' 'LBAL');
* create lookup table to exclude metadata;
*MBORRES MBSTRESC MBSTRESN MHDECOD
   MHENRTPT MHENTPT MHHLGT MHHLGTCD MHHLT
   MHHLTCD MHLLT MHTERM
PCORRES PCORRESU PCREFID PCSTRESC PCSTRESN
   VSORRES VSSTRESC VSSTRESN;
proc sql;
  create table clxmcall as
  select unique memname as dsn, name as var
  from sashelp.vcolumn where upcase(libname)
     = 'DSN' and memname in ('ADPCR' 'ADPRCS' 'ADBMK'
     'ADBMKS' 'ADCSF' 'ADCSFF')
and name
^in ('USUBJID' 'SUBJID' 'AETERM' 'LBORNRHI'
     'LBORNRLO' 'LBORRES' 'LBSTNRHI' 'LBSTNRLO' 'LBSTRESC'
     'LBSTRESN' 'AEHLGT' 'AEHLGTCD' 'AEHLT' 'AEHLTCD'
     'AELLT' 'AELLTCD' 'AEPTCD' 'AEDECOD'
'TRORRES' 'TRSTRESC' 'TRSTRESN' 'CMTRT' 'DAORRES'
     'DASTRESC' 'DASTRESN' 'ADT' 'AVAL' 'CHG' 'BASE'
     'AUCAVAL'  'DAY0VAL' 'PEAKVAL' 'TTPEAK' 'FCHG')
     and index(name, 'DT') = 0 and index(name, 'TM')
= 0 and index(name, 'SEQ') = 0 and index(name, 'DY') = 0
     order by memname, name;
quit;

* write to macro calling file;
data _null_;
set clxmcall;

file "\\analysis\dev\program\utility\codelist_ds_bmk.sas";
```

(Continued)

Example 7.1.1 (*Continued*): ADaM Codelist Dictionary

```
if _n_ = 1 then
put '%codev(dsn,'
dsn
','
var
', runnum=1)';
else
put '%codev(dsn,'
dsn
','
var
')';
run;

* metadata macro calls;
%inc "\\analysis\dev\program\utility\codelist_ds_bmk.sas";

ods html file="\\analysis\dev\program\utility\codelist_ds_bmk_&
   sysdate9..xls";
proc print data=codev noobs;
var _all_;
run;
ods html close;
```

The first partial screen shows the results of the generated macro calls for each dataset and variable combination. Once this SAS program is created, it is executed. This is an essential part to automate the process so the program is robust and dynamic for any number of datasets. In the first macro call, RUNNUM is set to 1 since this is the first dataset.

The second partial screen shows the Excel file with columns for each variable. The values listed in each row are in alphabetic sort order of all unique values. The column order is the same order as the macro calls in the SAS program. The columns represent the codelist dictionary for selected datasets and variables. In this Excel file, it is easy to review, search and confirm codelists.

Output

```
%codev(dsn,ADBMK , ABLFL , runnum=1)
%codev(dsn,ADBMK , ALSFL )
%codev(dsn,ADBMK , APERIOD )
%codev(dsn,ADBMK , APHASE )
%codev(dsn,ADBMK , APHASEN )
%codev(dsn,ADBMK , ARM )
%codev(dsn,ADBMK , ASSAYMET )
%codev(dsn,ADBMK , ASSAYNO )
%codev(dsn,ADBMK , AVISIT )
%codev(dsn,ADBMK , AVISITN )
%codev(dsn,ADBMK , BACKBS )
%codev(dsn,ADBMK , CCFL )
%codev(dsn,ADBMK , CMMT )
```

	A	B	C	D	E	F	G	H	I	J
1	ABLFL	ALSFL	APERIOD	APHASE	APHASEN	ARM	ASSAYMET	ASSAYNO	AVISIT	AVISITN
2	Y	Y	1	Phase1		1	MILLIPLEX MAP Human CD8+ T Cell Magnetic Bead Panel custom kit, PN HCD8MAG-15K	DR2A00	BASELINE	0
3			2	Phase2 Cohort1	2.1		MSD V-PLEX Plus Human Biomarker 40 Plex Kit, PN K15209G-4	DRA00B	DAY 7	7
4				Phase2 Cohort2	2.2		R&D Systems Human CD25/IL-2Ra Quantikine ELISA, PN DR2A00	ELLA-2	MONTH 12	14
5							R&D Systems Human IL-1Ra/IL-1F3 Quantikine ELISA, PN DRA00B	ELLA-F	MONTH 15	28
6							Simple Plex™ Human Ferritin Cartridge	HCD8MAG-15K	MONTH 18	90
7								K15209G-4	MONTH 24	180
8								K15209G-5	MONTH 3	270
9								ab108837	MONTH 6	360
10									MONTH 9	450
11									WEEK 2	540
12									WEEK 4	720

The example below compares differences in codelists. Codelists from ADaMs need to be a subset of the ADaM define specifications since the codelist in define.xml file may display extra codes that are within the codelist but not in ADaMs. Note that this example contains advanced macro programming to create and loop through records, dynamically creating macro calls for each ADaM and variable. Each intermediate dataset is then merged together in the same order as called so that codelists are grouped by ADaMs and variable order. Once all of the macro calls are created in a separate file, the file is included in the program to be executed. Proc IMPORT converts the codelist sheet in define spec to CODELIST1.

Example 7.1.2: ADaM Codelist Dictionary Difference

```
* Automatically compare dataset with define spec codelist;
libname dsn '\\analysis\data\adam' access=readonly;

options mprint mlogic symbolgen;

* read define spec;
* adams read id term;
proc import datafile="\\analysis\data\adam\xpt\define\define.
  xlsx"
      out=codelist1 (keep = id term) dbms=xlsx replace;
      sheet="codelists";
      getnames=yes;
run;

* adams;
data codelist (rename=id2=id);
length name $10. id2 $10.;
set codelist1;

name = scan(id, 1);
id2 = scan(id, 2);
drop id;
where id > '';
run;

proc sort data=codelist nodupkey out=clmcall1;
by name;
where name =: 'AD';
run;

data clmcall;
set clmcall1;

* for adams;
dsn=name;
```

(Continued)

Example 7.1.2 (*Continued*): ADaM Codelist Dictionary Difference

```
* sdtms;
*dsn=id;
*dsn=substr(id, 1, 2);
* include only matching domain names in codelist;
*where id in: ('AE' 'CM' 'CO' 'DA' 'DD' 'DM' 'DS' 'DV' 'EG' 'EX' 'FA'
   'HO' 'IE' 'IS' 'LB' 'MB' 'MH'
      'MI' 'MO' 'PC' 'PE' 'PR' 'QS' 'RS' 'SE' 'SS' 'SV' 'TA' 'TE' 'TI' 'TR'
   'TS' 'TU' 'TV' 'VS' 'XC');
*keep id dsn;

* note that LB is split into three versions LBAL, LBCY and LBLY;
if dsn='LB' then do;
dsn='LBAL'; output;
dsn='LBCY'; output;
dsn='LBLY'; output;
end;
else output;
run;

%macro ct_list(dsn=adsl, varn=race);
proc sql noprint;
* control term dataset for metadata checking;
select unique term into :mt_ctlist separated by ', ' from codelist
   where id=upcase("&varn");

* excludes missing values;
select unique &varn into :ds_ctlist separated by ', ' from dsn.&dsn
   where &varn > '';

create table dc as
select unique  "&dsn" as domain,
  compbl("&varn Codelist") as key_grp_vr length=50
  , "&ds_ctlist" as ds_ct label="Domain Codelist:" length=300
  , "&mt_ctlist" as mt_ct label="Control Terms Codelist:" length=300
```

(*Continued*)

Example 7.1.2 (*Continued*): ADaM Codelist Dictionary Difference

```
, case when "&ds_ctlist" ^= "&mt_ctlist" then 'Invalid Codelist'
else 'Valid Codelist' end as ctck label="&varn Codelist"
 from dsn.&dsn;
quit;

proc append base= dc_all data=dc force;
run;

%mend ct_list;

* write to macro calling file;
data _null_;
set clmcall;

file "\\analysis\dev\program\utility\codelist_dif.sas";
put '%ct_list(dsn='
dsn
', varn='
 id
')';
run;

* required to create dummy dataset for proc append;
data dc_all;
length domain $20. key_grp_vr $50. ds_ct $500. mt_ct $500. ctck $50.
define_update $20.;
run;

* metadata macro calls;
%inc "\\analysis\dev\program\utility\codelist_dif.sas";

proc sort data= dc_all nodupkey out=dc_all1;
by _all_;
run;
```

(*Continued*)

Example 7.1.2 (*Continued*): ADaM Codelist Dictionary Difference

```
data dc_all1;
set dc_all1;
if ctck = 'Valid Codelist' then define_update = 'n/a';
where domain > '';
run;

ods html file="\\analysis\dev\program\utility\codelist_
    dif_&sysdate9..xls";
proc print data=dc_all1 noobs;
var _all_;
run;
ods html close;
proc print; run;
```

Similar to the previous example, the first partial screen shows the results of the generated macro calls for each dataset and variable combination. Once this SAS program is created, it is executed. This is an essential part to automate the process so the program is robust and dynamic for any number of datasets.

In addition, the second partial screen shows the Excel file with columns for each variable. The values listed in each row are in alphabetic sort order of all unique values. The column order is the same order as the macro calls in the SAS program. The columns represent the codelist dictionary for selected datasets and variables. In this Excel file, it is easy to review, search and confirm codelists. CTCK displays VALID or INVALID CODELIST for each ADaM and variable. For INVALID CODELIST rows, lists DS_CAT from ADaM and MT_CAT from define spec can be compared and updated.

Output

```
%ct_list(dsn=ADAE , varn=KREL30FL )
%ct_list(dsn=ADDA , varn=PARAM )
%ct_list(dsn=ADEFF , varn=PARAM )
%ct_list(dsn=ADEX , varn=PARAM )
%ct_list(dsn=ADIS , varn=PARAM )
%ct_list(dsn=ADLB , varn=PARAM )
%ct_list(dsn=ADMB , varn=PARAM )
%ct_list(dsn=ADPCR , varn=PARAM )
%ct_list(dsn=ADPCRS , varn=PARAM )
%ct_list(dsn=ADQS , varn=PARAM )
%ct_list(dsn=ADRS , varn=PARAM )
%ct_list(dsn=ADSAF , varn=PARAM )
%ct_list(dsn=ADSL , varn=SEX )
%ct_list(dsn=ADTR , varn=PARAM )
%ct_list(dsn=ADTTE , varn=PARAM )
```

	A	B	C	D	E	F
1	domain	key_grp_vr	ds_ct	mt_ct	ctck	define_update
2	ADAE	KREL30FL Codelist	N, Y	N, Y	Valid Codelist	n/a
3	ADDA	PARAM Codelist	CD3 Cells, CD4 Cells, CD4/CD8 Ratio, CD8 Cells, Central Memory Cells, Dispensed Amount, Effector Cells, Effector Memory Cells, Infused Amount, Interferon Gamma, KTE-C19 Delivery, KTE-C19 Time from Leukapheresis to Delivery at Site, Manufacturing Dose Produced, Naive Cells, Patient Weight at IP admin	% B Cells of Viable Leukocytes (%), Absolute Basophils Count (10^9/L), Absolute Eosinophils Count (10^9/L), Absolute Monocyte Count (10^9/L), Alanine Aminotransferase (U/L), Albumin (g/L), Alkaline Phosphatase (U/L), Antibody Test (pg/mL), Aspartate Aminotransferase (U/L), Basophils/Leukocytes (%),	Invalid Codelist	
4	ADEFF	PARAM Codelist	Best Overall Resp. by Cent. Read Per. 01, Best Overall Resp. by Cent. Read Per. 02, Best Overall Response by Inv. Per. 01, Best Overall Response by Inv. Per. 02, First Obj. Response in Per. 01 by Central Read, First Obj. Response in Per. 01 by Investigator, First Obj. Response in Per. 02 by Central	% B Cells of Viable Leukocytes (%), Absolute Basophils Count (10^9/L), Absolute Eosinophils Count (10^9/L), Absolute Monocyte Count (10^9/L), Alanine Aminotransferase (U/L), Albumin (g/L), Alkaline Phosphatase (U/L), Antibody Test (pg/mL), Aspartate Aminotransferase (U/L), Basophils/Leukocytes (%).	Invalid Codelist	

7.2 CODELIST AND VALUE-LEVEL UPPERCASE

Codelist and value-level uppercase checks confirm no lower or proper case controlled terms. Proc SQL compares the variable with UPCASE() to assign BAD_VALUE 1 for any mismatch. DCA identifies which records fail, and DCB identifies the overall check. All SEX values are in uppercase.

Example 7.2.1: Codelist and Value-Level Uppercase

```
proc sql;
  create table dca as
  select a.usubjid, a.sex,
  case when ^(sex = upcase(sex)) then 1
  else . end as bad_value label='FAIL: NOT Upcase SEX'
  from adsl as a;

create table dcb as
select unique 'ADSL' as domain,
  compbl("SUBJECTID / SEX") as key_grp_vr length=50
  , case when count(bad_value) = 0 then 'PASS: All are Upper Case'
  else 'FAIL: At Least one Not Upper Case' end as dc_rslt
    label="Data Check Results For:" length=75
  from dca;
quit;
```

The results display PASS that all sex values are all uppercase.

Output

Obs	domain	key_grp_vr	dc_rslt
1	ADSL	SUBJECTID / SEX	PASS: All are Upper Case

SUMMARY

This chapter provides examples of codelist dictionary compliance checks for SDTMs and ADaMs. While standardized controlled terms greatly facilitate review and analysis of the data, data value checks are still required since there are many opportunities for unexpected programming or data errors in the SDTM and ADaM creation process.

Appendix

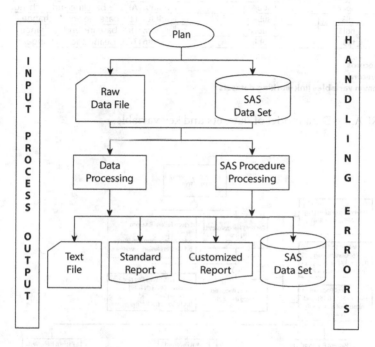

FIGURE A.1 Anatomy of a SAS program.

Type	Dataset	Common Variables					Description/Extracted Variables
1:1	analyvar	usubjid	subjid	cohort			Base dataset
	cs1rand	usubjid					Cohort and treatment
	cs1rand2	usubjid					Cohort and treatment
	_dose	usubjid					Dosing variables
1:M	_pk2	usubjid			pk_code	drawdt	PK Draw variables from excel file
	_pkcrf	usubjid			pkrefid		PK variables from CRF
	_dday	usubjid		cohort		daydt	Dose Day
	_fdday	usubjid					First Dose Day
	_ndose	usubjid				pkdtf	Number of dose days
	_apoc3		subjid			visitdtn	APOC3 baseline and % change
	_ldl3		subjid			visitdtn	LDL baseline and % change
	_hdl3		subjid			visitdtn	HDL baseline and % change
	_tg3		subjid			visitdtn	TG baseline and % change
1:1 records							
1:M records							
Common variables link working datasets							

FIGURE A.2 Data model of datasets and key variables.

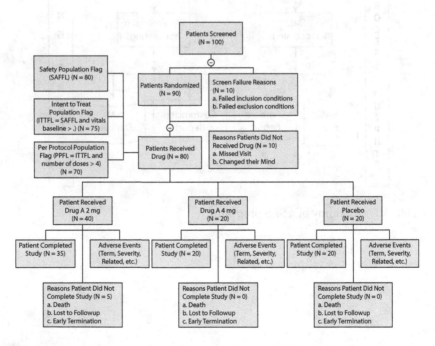

FIGURE A.3 Subject disposition tree from enrollment to study completion.

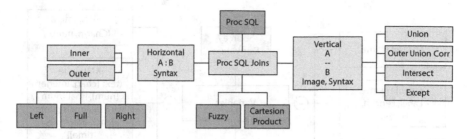

FIGURE A.4   Proc SQL joins mind map.

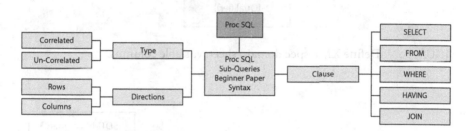

FIGURE A.5   Proc SQL subqueries mind map.

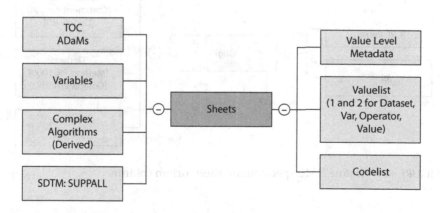

FIGURE A.6   Define XML spec domain sheets.

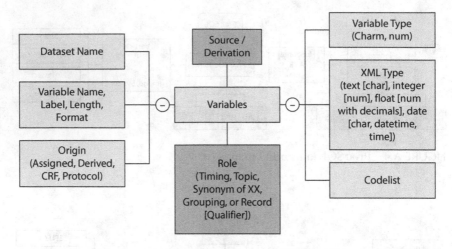

FIGURE A.7   Define XML spec domain sheet: variable columns.

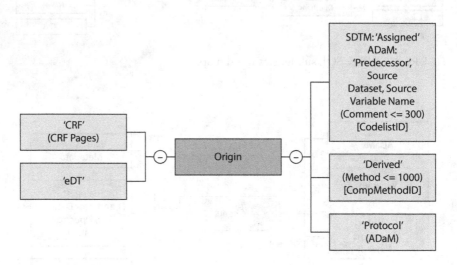

FIGURE A.8   Define XML spec domain sheet: origin column.

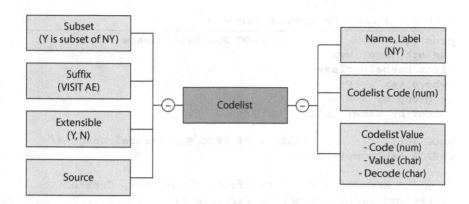

FIGURE A.9   Define XML spec codelist columns.

TABLE A.1   Four Key Metadata/Dictionary Datasets

Category	Description	PROC SQL: Dictionary Table	PROC SQL or DATA Step: SASHelp View
1. Dictionaries	Category of files: Catalogs, etc.	Dictionary. dictionaries	sashelp.vdctnry
2. Members	List of SAS libraries and data sets	Dictionary. members	sashelp.vmember
3. Table	List of data sets and columns	Dictionary. tables	sashelp.vtable
4. Columns	List of columns and attributes	Dictionary. columns	sashelp.vcolumn

TABLE A.2   Proc SQL Productive Summary Sheet

```
proc sql;                    /* PROC SQL Basic Usage */
 select name, sex
 from sashelp.class
 where sex = 'F'
 < group by > < having >
 order by name; quit;

PROC SQL;          /* Anatomy of PROC SQL General Usage */
CREATE table mytable as

/* Eight Benefits: Validate/Create View/Table, Create/
Alter/Update/Insert/Delete Variable */

/* 1. Four Components: a. SELECT, b. FROM, c. WHERE,
 d. ORDER */

A. SELECT name, sex

 /* 2. Four selecting columns options:
        a. ',' to separate columns
        b. label=' ' format= $10. length=10 to add attributes
        c. '*' to select all columns
        d. distinct to select unique columns */

 /* 3. Six creating columns options:
        a. functions ex. init((age + 150)/10) as myage
        b. summary function ex. max(height,
           weight) as maxval
        c. summary function ex. ((weight/sum(weight))*100) as
           wpercent
        d. constant ex. 'my home' as myhome
        e. character expression ex. city || ',' || state as
           address
        f. select case when age < 13 then 1 else 0 end as
           agegrp */
```

(Continued)

TABLE A.2 (*Continued*)   Proc SQL Productive Summary Sheet

```
/* 6. Five macro variable creating options:
      a. into : to store one value in one macro variable
      b. into : separated by to store multiple values
      c. into : - : to create multiple macro variables
      d. summary function into: to create
         one macro variable
      e. select-case into:  to create
         one macro variable */

B. FROM sashelp.class as class, Mylib.students as students
/* Four join options: inner matching/outer LEFT/FULL/
RIGHT JOIN */
/* FROM <DS1> <FULL JOIN> <DS2>  ON <DS1.VAR1> = <DS2.
VAR2> */

C. WHERE class.name = students.name and class.sex = 'F'
/* 4. Four subsetting options:
      a. direct variable using where clause
      b. calculated variable using where clause
      c. function, ex. index(name, 'B') using where clause
      d. summary function, ex. sum(sales) > 0 using
         having clause */

/* 5. Two subquery options:
      a. one value returned
      b. multiple values returned with <Variable> < IN Operator>
(SELECT <Variable> FROM <Table> WHERE <Condition Expression>) */

D. ORDER by name
/* Two sorting options: order/group by calculated, desc */
; QUIT;
```

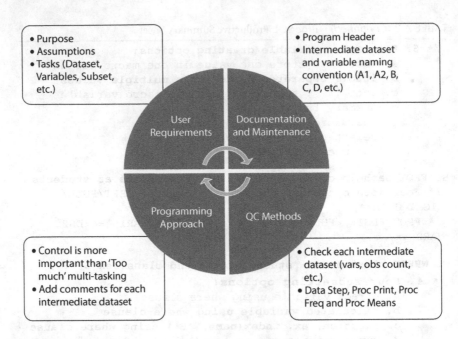

- Purpose
- Assumptions
- Tasks (Dataset, Variables, Subset, etc.)

- Program Header
- Intermediate dataset and variable naming convention (A1, A2, B, C, D, etc.)

User Requirements

Documentation and Maintenance

Programming Approach

QC Methods

- Control is more important than 'Too much' multi-tasking
- Add comments for each intermediate dataset

- Check each intermediate dataset (vars, obs count, etc.)
- Data Step, Proc Print, Proc Freq and Proc Means

FIGURE A.10   Effective unit testing concepts for proc SQL.

TABLE A.3   One-Proc Away Using Proc Tabulate: Knowing Your Row and Column Options

Row Options Flexible Structure Ex. Key Variables & Descriptive Stats	Column Options Fixed Structure Ex. By Treatment Groups	All
Numeric	Numeric	
Or	Or	
Character Variables	Character Variables	
Categorical (Unique values – N, %)	Categorical (Unique values – N, %)	
Or	Or	
Continuous Variables (Descriptive Statistics – N, NMISS, MIN, Q1, Q3, MAX)	Continuous Variables (Descriptive Statistics – N, NMISS, MIN, Q1, Q3, MAX)	
Control Order w/ PreLoadFormat/Group Formats	Control Order w/ PreLoadFormat/Group Formats	
Or	Or	
Non-Missing/Missing	Non-Missing/Missing	
All,	Concatenate	
Concatenate	or	
or	Nest Variables	
Nest Variables		

Note: One Record per USUBJID based on Condition and/or By Variables.

TABLE A.4   Raw Data to SDTMs to ADaMs Compliance Checklist

SDTM Classes

ADaMs from SDTMs from Raw Data

- **Example Macros**: %var_def, %excel2sas, %m_empty_dataset, %sort_order, %dtc, %dtc2dt, %dt_impute, %dt_dur, %bl_flg, %chgbl, %maxchar, %xxseq, %suppxx, %study_day, %comp_ds, %m_codelist_fmt, %merg_suppxx, %split_coval, %avisit_wn, %dtype_avg, %code_v, %code_dif, %scan_log, %p21_chks, %one_mean, %one_freq, %sql_grp_stats, %qc_tlfs, %ds_vitals
- **P21 Data Issues**: a. invalid Raw data such as dates, b. Duplicate Records exist, c. invalid Codelists such as RACEOTH.
- **CDISC Rule Issues**: a. invalid Structure such as incorrect order or missing required var, b. invalid ISO 8601 format, c. inconsistent Multiple related vars such as DTC and DY vars.

Special Domains – One record per USUBJID, Required

- Demog (DM vs SC)/(ADSL)
- Comments (CO)
- Inclusion and Exclusion (IE) vs Trial Inclusion (TI) vs Deviation (DV)

Trial Design – Required, Excel metadata

- Trial Elements (TE), Trial Arms (TA), Trial Visits (TV)
- Subject Elements (SE), Subject Visits (SV)

Interventions – One record per USUBJID, Timestamp, Term

- Occurrence Structure Model (OCCRS)
- ConMeds (CM)/(ADCM)
- Exposure (EX – required vs EC vs DC)/(ADEX)

Events – One record per USUBJID, Timestamp, Event

- Occurrence Structure Model (OCCRS)
- Adverse Events (AE vs CS)/(ADAE)
- Disposition (DS – required)
- Medical History (MH)

Findings – One record per USUBJID, Timestamp, Finding

- Basic Data Structure Model (BDS)
- Labs (LB)/(ADLB)
- Questionnaire (QS)/(ADQS)
- Vital Signs (VS)/(ADVS)

Relationships/SUPP Qual – One record per USUBJID, IDVARVAL

- Findings About (FA) – By usubjid fatestcd faobj visitnum fatptref fatptnum;
- Related Records (RELREC) – By usubjid idvarval relid;
- Supplemental Qualifier (SUPPXX) – By usubjid idvarval qnam;

TABLE A.5   Clinical Study and CDISC Compliance Checklist

Milestone Task

Database Lock Process
- Cutoff date, Snapshot date
- Database acceptance checks

Data Handling Process
- Common derivations, Missing values
- Imputation rules

Case Report Form (CRF)
- Blankcrf.pdf (annotated w/bookmark table of contents)

Metadata Files for Data-Driven Process
- Map Raw to SDTMs, to ADaMs Mapping
- Map Titles and Footnotes to TLFs

Controlled Terminology
- Control Terms, Value-Level Metadata
- Lookup Tables

SDTMs from Raw Data Mapping
- Programming Style, No hard-coding, Clean Logs
- Required Domains (TA, DM, EX, DS)
- Total # pts: IE >= DM >= EX >= DV/AE/DS
- Max Character Variable Lengths (%maxchar)
- Pinnacle 21 Report and In-house checks
- QC, QA and Reviewer's Guide
- XPTs, DEFINE.XML with hyperlinks, Pinnacle 21 report

ADaMs from SDTMs Mapping
- Programming Style, No hard-coding, Clean Logs
- Derived PARAMCD and Records
- Traceable to SDTMs (SRCDOM, SRCVAR)
- Pinnacle 21 Report and In-house checks
- QC, QA and Reviewer's Guide
- XPTs, DEFINE.XML with hyperlinks, Pinnacle 21 report

Tables, Lists and Figures from ADaMs
- Annotated table shells, titles, footnotes
- Programming Style, No hard-coding, Clean Logs
- Big N, QC and DEFINE.XML
- Log Dates: SDTMs <= ADaMs <= TLFs
- Clear all data and reporting issues

Statistical Results
- Demographics and Baseline Tables, P-value
- Primary and Secondary Tables, P-value
- Adverse Events Tables, P-value
- Protocol Compliance Tables, P-value

TABLE A.6   Pinnacle 21 Issues Checklist

Pinnacle 21 C and E (Data Packages)

SDTM IG version # 3.2 (MedDRA 21.0, WHO Drug xx)
- DDT with English Vars Derivations (%excel2sas)
- Common and Domain P21 E Issues
- Duplicate Records Check (by _all_, by key variables)
- 5 Channel Compliance Checks: Unit, Multiple Vars/Datasets, New Vars, Protocol Comp., Metadata/Data Transfer Metrics

ADaM IG version # 1.0
- DDT with English Vars Derivations (%excel2sas)
- Common and Domain P21 E Issues
- Duplicate Records Check (by _all_, by key variables)
- 5 Channel Compliance Checks: Unit, Multiple Vars/Datasets, New Vars, Protocol Comp., Metadata/Data Transfer Metrics

SDTM Metadata Repository (DEFINE.XLS)
- Prepopulate sheets with XPT or P21 E validation metadata
- Codelist Dictionary for all SDTMs (%code_v)
- Prepopulate CRF Page # with P21E validation

ADaM Metadata Repository (DEFINE.XLS)
- Prepopulate sheets with XPT or P21 E validation metadata
- Codelist Dictionary for all ADaMs

Controlled Terminology (SDTM # 2017-12-22, ADaM # 2017-09-29)
- Codelist Differences to assure all codes are in DEFINE.XLS (%code_dif)
- Decode Text, ex. RACE
- For Multiple Values only instead of Single Value, ex. CRIT1
- Sponsor-specific codelists, non 'CXX'

Value-Level Metadata, ex. PARAMCD
- Codelist Differences to assure all codes are in DEFINE.XLS (%code_dif)
- Shared and ADaM specific Value-Level Metadata
- AVAL/C, Where PARAM/CD = 'XXX', List of PARAM/CD values

Reviewer Guides (CSDRG, ADRG)
- Prepopulate P21 E Issues section with P21 E Validation and Explanations
- List of Explanations for Duplicate Records

DEFINE.XML version # 2.0
- Manual WordPad updates to address final P21 E issues, ex. alias
- P21 E and P21 C Issues Minimized (SDTM, ADaM and CT version #)
- Internal reference links (Dataset, Variable, CT, VLM)
- CSDRG and ADRG Reviewer Guide links
- ACRF Page # Links for each variable, XPTs, Complexalgorithms

TABLE A.7   Pinnacle 21 Define Spec to Define XML Checklist

Define Spec Sheet Columns
See P21-MappingSpec-Template-Instructions_V3.xls

Study Sheet Columns (Mostly Manual entry unless from P21 E)
- Value – Project and Study metadata

Datasets Sheet Columns (Mostly from P21 C)
- Dataset, Description, Class, Structure, Purpose, Key Variables, Repeating, Reference data and Comment

Variables Sheet Columns (Mostly from P21 C)
- Order, Dataset, Variable, Label, Type, Length, Mandatory, Role
- CRF Page # in P21 E, For **Origin=CRF** only, from acrf even if assigned
- Codelist – DOMAIN, MEDDRA, (Match Control Terms)
- Origin – Assigned, Derived or CRF
- Method – populated for all Origin = 'Derived', ex. AE.AESEQ
- Comment – populated for all Origin ^='Derived', ex. AE.STUDYID

ValueLevel Sheet Columns
- Order, Dataset, Variable, **Where Clause**, Data type, Length, Significant digits, Format, Mandatory, **Codelist**, Origin, Pages, Method, Predecessor, Value level comment, Join comment
- Use P21E validation report if not too many standards

Whereclauses Sheet Columns
- **For each matching ValueLevel. Where clause**, Create row – ID, Dataset, Variable, Comparator, Value
- One to one record with ValueLevel

Codelist Sheet Columns
- **For each matching Variable. Codelist**, Create row – ID, Name, NCI codelist code, Data type, Order, Term, NCI term code, Decoded value (if different from Term value)
- P21E creates codelist for up to 40 unique values, Need to manually add code if on CRF but not in data

Dictionaries Sheet Columns
- ID – One MEDDRA row

Methods Sheet Columns
- For each matching Variable. Method and Variables. Origin ='Derived', ex. AE.AESEQ, Create row – ID, Name, Type, Description

Comments Sheet Columns
- For each matching Variables. Comment and Variables. Origin ^='Derived', ex. AE.STUDYID, Create row – ID, Description

Documents Sheet Columns
- One row for each file to link acrf.pdf, csdrg.pdf, length_derivations.pdf

TABLE A.8   Useful Tips for Processing Excel Files

a. To compare two columns, create a third column using the IF() function with 'Match' or 'Not Match' values.

```
IF(Q25=W25, "Match", "Not Match")
```

b. To compare two columns as from 3rd position for qc program name, create a third column using the IF() function with 'Match' or 'Not Match' values.

```
IF(Q25=MID(W25, 3, 20), "Match", "Not Match")
```

c. Sometimes in the Excel file there will be fields entered by Alt+Enter keys which will put the data in more than one line within a cell. To remove these linefeed '0A'x hidden characters, which can cause errors in macro programs, apply the =CLEAN(A1) function in a second excel column. To remove linefeeds within variables, apply the TRANSLATE(LABEL, " ", '0A'x) function in the program.

d. To convert an XLSX excel file with multiple sheets into intermediate datasets, apply the code below. PROC SQL creates a metadata dataset from accessing the MYXLSX libname with macro variables SNAMLIST to contain list of all sheets and N for total number of sheets. Next in the do loop, for each sheet, PROC IMPORT creates dataset with the same sheet name. Use DBMS=XLSX for XLSX file types or DBMS=EXCEL for XLS file types. The option SCANTEXT=YES can be applied for SAS to read the entire column and use the length of the longest string found as the variable length.

```
libname myxlsx 'c:\ddt' access=readonly;

proc sql;
create table spec_meta as select * from dictionary.
tables where libname="MYXLS";
select memname into :snamlist separated by '*' from spec_
meta;
select count(memname) into :n from spec_meta;
quit;
%put &snamlist;
%put &n;

%macro m1;
%do i=1 %to &n;
%let var=%scan(&snamlist, &i, *);

proc import out= work.%substr(&var,1,%length(&var)-1)
datafile= "c:\ddt\SDTM Metadata.xlsx"
dbms=xlsx replace;
sheet="&var";
getnames=yes;
run;
%end;
%mend m1;
%m1
```

(Continued)

TABLE A.8 (*Continued*)   Useful Tips for Processing Excel Files

---

e. To convert a dataset into an excel file, apply the code below. See more examples of Proc EXPORT in chapter 7.

```
PROC EXPORT data=test.define.test
    outfile='c:\myfiles\class'
    dbms=EXCEL;
RUN;
```

f. To create a macro variable containing a list of variables in order of DM specification from DM sheet in excel file, apply the code below which will create the correct syntax to reference excel variable names. The following data step applies the macro variable in a RETAIN statement which controls the variables in DM.

```
proc sql;
    select unique "'" || compbl(name) || "'n" into
:dmvrlst separated by " "
    from sashelp.vcolumn where upcase(libname) = 'WORK' and
upcase(memname) = 'DM' order by monotonic();
quit;
%let gbaylst = &dmvrlst;
%put & dmvrlst

data dm;
  retain & dmvrlst;
  set dm;
run;
```

References

FDA DOCUMENTATION

Electronic Common Technical Document (eCTD). https://www.fda.gov/drugs/
    electronic-regulatory-submission-and-review/electronic-common-technical-
    document-ectd.
Guidance Documents. https://www.fda.gov/drugs/guidances-drugs/newly-
    added-guidance-documents.
Study Data Technical Conformance Guide. https://www.fda.gov/media/88173/
    download.

INDUSTRY DOCUMENTATION

CDISC. https://www.cdisc.org/.
Case Report Tabulation Data Definition Specification (define.xml). https://
    www.cdisc.org/system/files/all/standard_category/application/pdf/crt_
    ddspecification1_0_0.pdf.
ICH. http://www.ich.org/products/guidelines.html.
Pinnacle 21. https://www.pinnacle21.com/.

ARTICLES AND PAPERS

Abousahl-Chaunu, Isabelle. 'Standards for the Management of Clinical Trial
    Data, Why Are They Needed, What Is Needed?', *Proceedings of PhUSE* 2013.
Amoruccio, Vincent. 'Could Have, Would Have, Should Have! Adopting Good
    Programming Standards, Not Practices, to Survive an Audit', *Proceedings
    of PharmaSUG* 2012.
Chang, Christina, Chang, Kyle. 'SDTM Electronic Submissions to FDA:
    Guidelines and Best Practices', *Proceedings of PharmaSUG* 2015.
Chen, Huei-Ling. 'ADaM Dataset Checking Toolkit', *Proceedings of PharmaSUG*
    2010.
Coulson, Susan Fehrer, Coulson, Kevin R. 'Mission Possible: Your Assignment Is
    to Validate Output for a Study', *Proceedings of PharmaSUG* 2013.
Dalvi, Amita. 'Clinical Study Report Review: Statistician's Approach', *Proceedings
    of PharmaSUG* 2014.
Dey, Mei, Peers, Diane. 'Delivering a Quality CDISC Compliant Accelerated
    Submission Using an Outsourced Model', *Proceedings of PharmaSUG* 2016.

DiIorio, Frank, Abolafia, Jeff. 'From CRF Data to Define.Xml: Going "End to End" with Metadata', *Proceedings of PharmaSUG 2007*.

DiIorio Frank, Abolafi, Jeffrey. 'Results-Level Metadata: What, How, and Why', *Proceedings of PharmaSUG 2016*.

Gupta, Sunil. *Sharpening Your SAS Skills*, CRC Press, 2005.

Gupta, Sunil. *'Standards for Clinical Data Quality and Compliance Checks'*, Pharmaceutical Programming, 2008, Data Basics, Society for Clinical Data Management, Winter 2008 newsletter.

Gupta, Sunil. 'Clinical-Data Acceptance Testing Procedure', *Proceedings of the SAS Global Forum 2008*.

Gupta, Sunil. 'Ready to Become Really Productive Using PROC SQL?', *Proceedings of the SAS Global Forum 2013*.

Gupta, Sunil. 'Something for Nothing? Adding Group Descriptive Statistics Using PROC SQL Subqueries', *Proceedings of the SAS Global Forum 2013*.

Gupta, Sunil. *'How Cloud-Based Tools Can Help with FDA Compliance'*, Life Science Leader, August 30, 2013, https://www.lifescienceleader.com/doc/how-cloud-based-tools-can-help-with-fda-compliance-0001.

Gupta, Sunil. *Sharpening Your Advanced SAS Skills*, CRC Press, 2015.

Gupta, Sunil, Lafler, Kirk, 'Solving Business Problems with the SQL Procedure', *Proceedings of the SAS Global Forum 21*.

Jehl, Genevieve. 'Clinical Database Acceptance: What Statistical Review Checks Are Necessary to Validate a Database?', *Proceedings of PharmaSUG 2009*.

Lin, Qin, Kelly, Tim. 'Standard SAS Macros for Standard Date/Time Processing', *Proceedings of NESUG 2006*.

Marchand, Cedric, Tinazz, Angelo. 'What Auditors Want', *PhUSE 2016*.

Nguyen, Sandra VanPelt. 'Validating define.xml: Tools, Trials, and Tribulations', *Proceedings of PharmaSUG 2011*.

Santema, Michael, Xie, Fagen. 'How to STRIP Your Data: Five Go-To Steps to Assure Data Quality', *Proceedings of SGF 2016*.

Sarmukadam, Sneha, Sawant, Sandeep. 'Programmer's Safety Kit: Important Points to Remember While Programming or Validating Safety Tables', *Proceedings of PhamaSUG 2012*.

Silva, Greg. 'CODEBOOK: Taking Another Look at Your Data', *Proceedings of SUGI 25*.

Shilling, Brian. 'The 5 Most Important Clinical SAS Programming Validation Steps', *Proceedings of NESUG 10*.

Sirichenko, Sergiy, DiGiantomasso, Michael, Collopy, Travis. 'Usage of Pinnacle 21 Community Toolset 2.1.1 for Clinical Programmers', *Proceedings of PharmaSUG 2016*.

Sirichenko, Sergiy, Kanevsky, Max. 'The Most Common Issues in Submission Data', *Proceedings of PharmaSUG 2015*.

Tinazzi, Angelo, Colombini, Sonia, Comarella, Lisa, Zanus, Marta. 'Is Your Output Telling the Truth? Tips and Tricks in Verifying SAS Outputs', *Proceedings of PhUSE 2006*.

Xia, Jeff, Xie, Lugang. 'A Well-Formatted and Easy-to-Navigate Solution for Submitting SAS Source Code in NDA Submission', *Proceedings of WUSS* 2016.

Xu, Linfeng, Gupta, Sunil. 'Saving QC Time for Production Tables', *Proceedings of PharmaSUG* 2007.

Zhong, Wayne. 'Building and Customizing a CDISC Compliance and Data Quality Application', *Proceedings of WUSS* 2015.

Index

Note: Page numbers in italic and bold refer to figures and tables, respectively.

Printed in the United States
by Baker & Taylor Publisher Services

Printed in the United States
by Baker & Taylor Publisher Services